Weight Loss with the Mediterranean Diet

Turn a day-by-day Diet into a Lifetime Habit

Sasha Merianelli

Table of Contents

Pizza Pockets

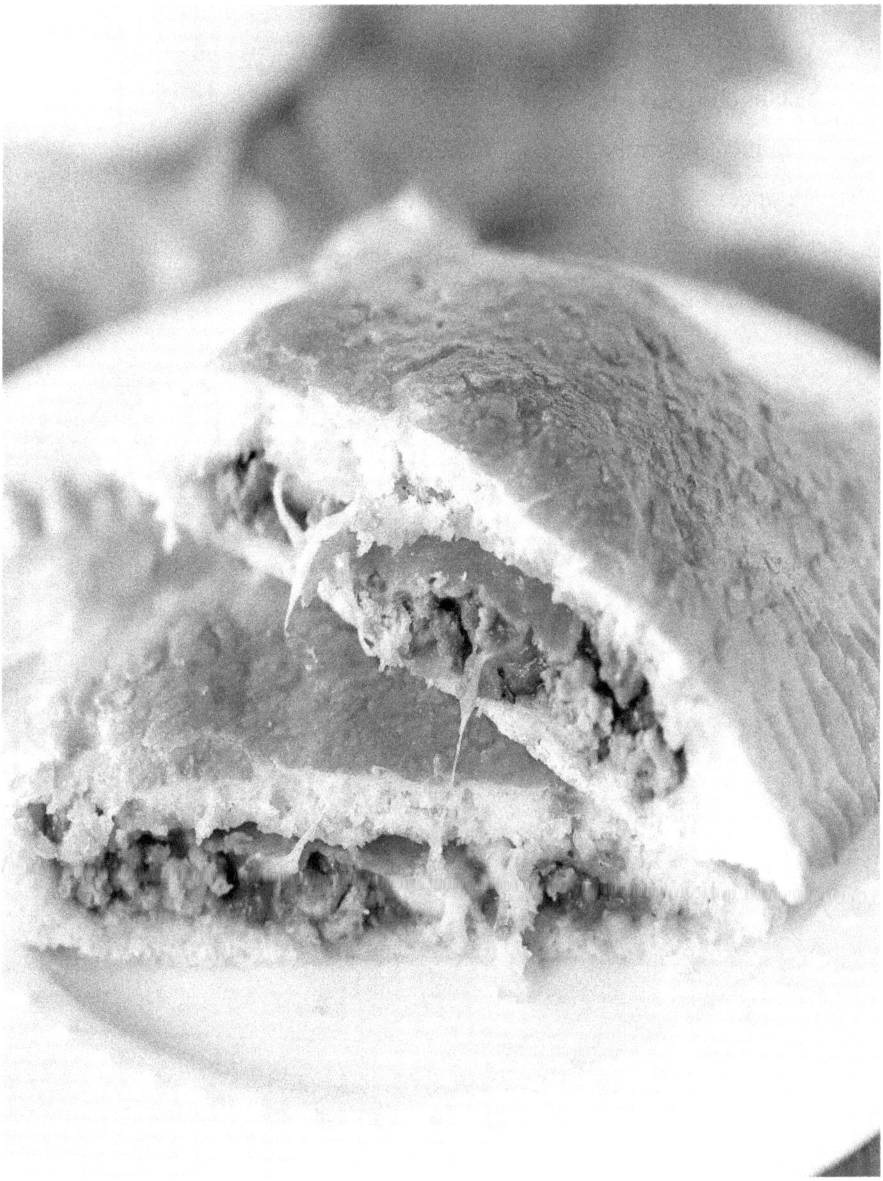

Prep time:

10 minutes | Cook time: 0 minutes | Serves 2

Ingredients

½ cup tomato sauce

½ teaspoon oregano

½ teaspoon garlic powder

½ cup chopped black olives

2 canned artichoke hearts, drained and chopped

2 ounces (57 g) pepperoni, chopped

½ cup shredded Mozzarella cheese

1 whole-wheat pita, halved

Direction

1. In a medium bowl, stir together the tomato sauce, oregano, and garlic powder.
2. Add the olives, artichoke hearts, pepperoni, and cheese. Stir to mix.
3. Spoon the mixture into the pita halves and serve.

Per Serving

Calories: 375 | fat: 23.5g | protein: 17.1g | carbs: 27.1g | fiber: 6.1g | sodium: 1080mg

Mushroom-Pesto Baked Pizza

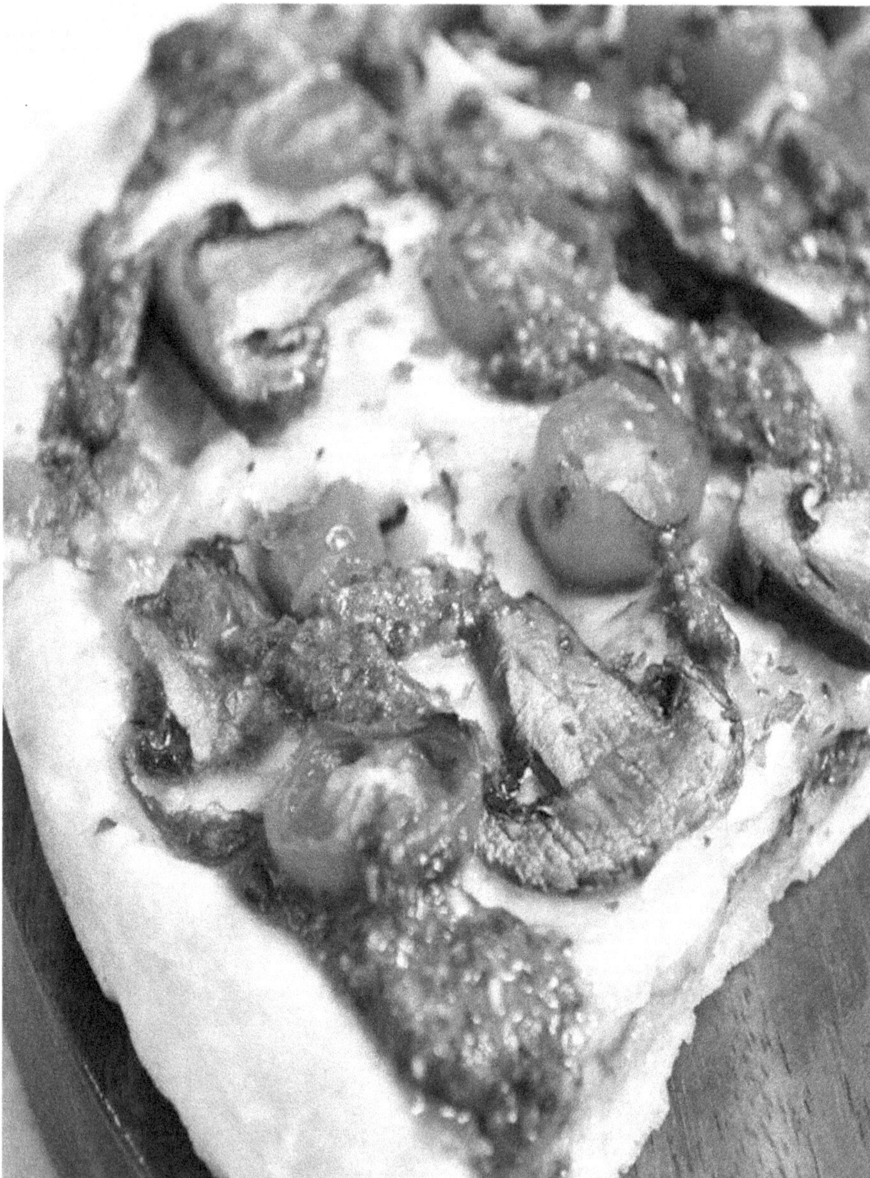

Prep time:

5 minutes | Cook time: 15 minutes | Serves 2

Ingredients

1 teaspoon extra-virgin olive oil

½ cup sliced mushrooms

½ red onion, sliced

Salt and freshly ground black pepper

¼ cup store-bought pesto sauce

2 whole-wheat flatbreads

¼ cup shredded Mozzarella cheese

Direction

1. Preheat the oven to 350ºF (180ºC).
2. In a small skillet, heat the oil over medium heat. Add the mushrooms and onion, and season with salt and pepper. Sauté for 3 to 5 minutes until the onion and mushrooms begin to soften.
3. Spread 2 tablespoons of pesto on each flatbread.
4. Divide the mushroom-onion mixture between the two flatbreads. Top each with 2 tablespoons of cheese.
5. Place the flatbreads on a baking sheet and bake for 10 to 12 minutes until the cheese is melted and bubbly. Serve warm.

Per Serving

Calories: 348 | fat: 23.5g | protein: 14.2g | carbs: 28.1g | fiber: 7.1g | sodium: 792mg

Tuna and Hummus Wraps

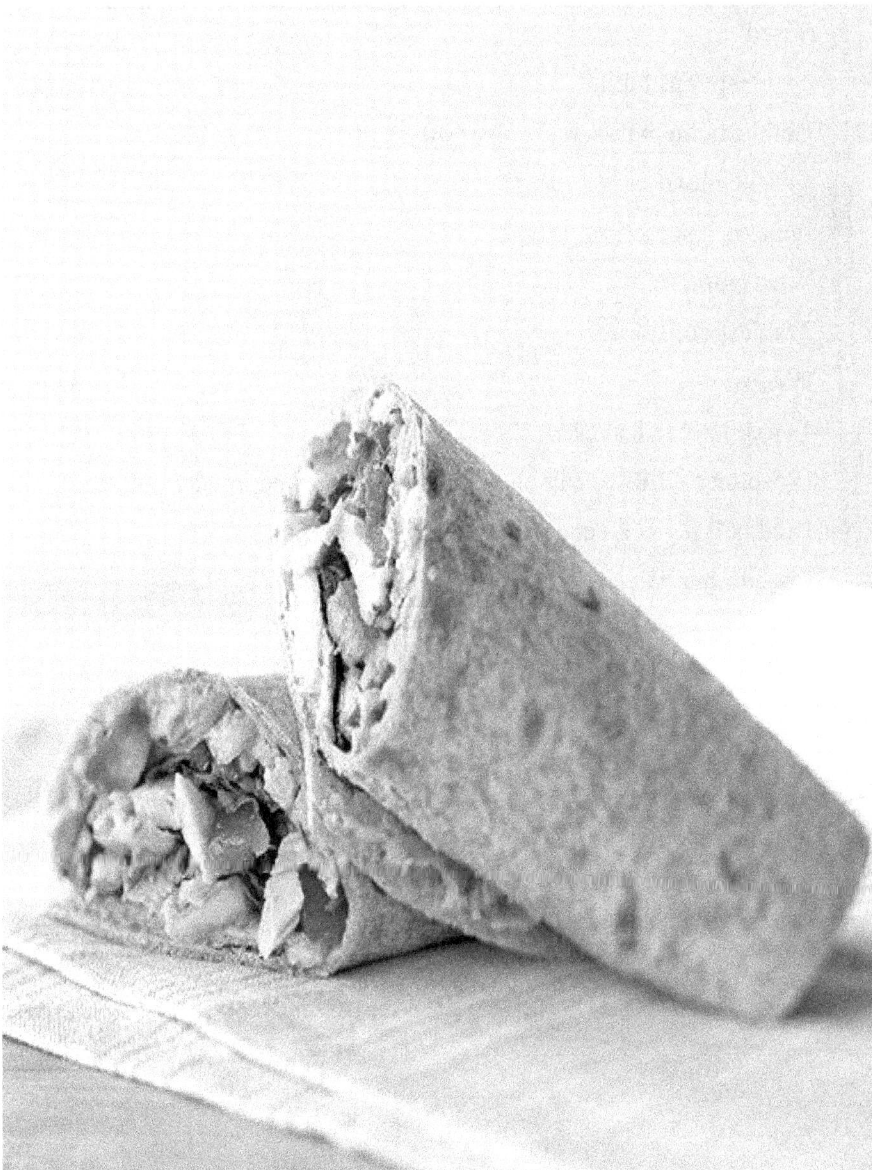

Prep time:

10 minutes | Cook time: 0 minutes | Serves 2

Ingredients

Hummus:

1 cup from 1 (15-ounce / 425-g) can low-sodium chickpeas, drained and rinsed

2 tablespoons tahini

1 tablespoon extra-virgin olive oil

1 garlic clove

Juice of ½ lemon

¼ teaspoon salt

2 tablespoons water

Wraps:

4 large lettuce leaves

1 (5-ounce / 142-g) can chunk light tuna packed in water, drained

1 red bell pepper, seeded and cut into strips

1 cucumber, sliced

Direction

Make the Hummus

1. In a blender jar, combine the chickpeas, tahini, olive oil, garlic, lemon juice, salt, and water. Process until smooth. Taste and adjust with additional lemon juice or salt, as needed.

Make the Wraps

2. On each lettuce leaf, spread 1 tablespoon of hummus, and divide the tuna among the leaves. Top each with several strips of red pepper and cucumber slices.
3. Roll up the lettuce leaves, folding in the two shorter sides and rolling away from you, like a burrito. Serve immediately.

Per Serving

Calories: 192 | fat: 5.1g | protein: 26.1g | carbs: 15.1g | fiber: 4.1g | sodium: 352mg

Chickpea Lettuce Wraps

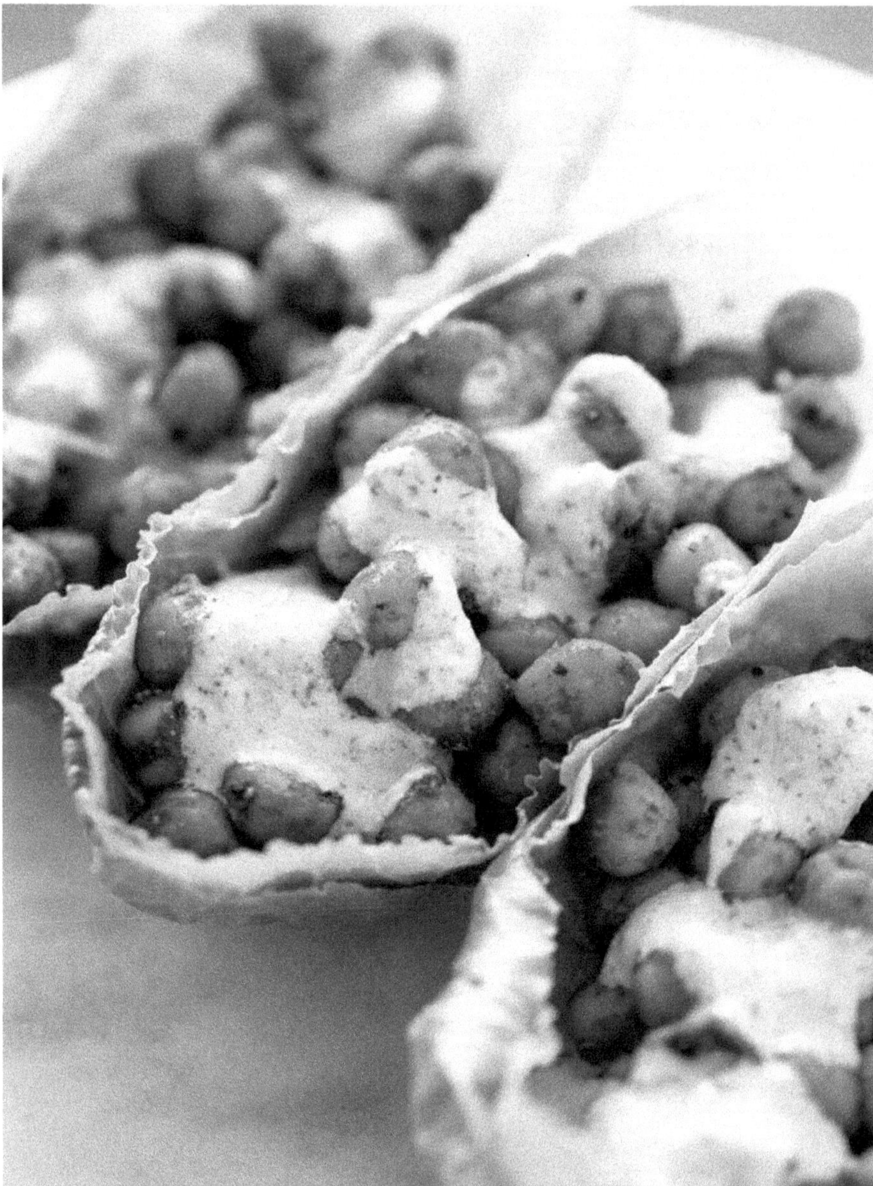

Prep time:

15 minutes | Cook time: 0 minutes | Serves 2

Ingredients

1 (15-ounce / 425-g) can chickpeas, drained and rinsed well

1 celery stalk, diced

½ shallot, minced

1 green apple, cored and diced

3 tablespoons tahini (sesame paste)

2 teaspoons freshly squeezed lemon juice

1 teaspoon raw honey

1 teaspoon Dijon mustard Dash salt

Filtered water, to thin

4 romaine lettuce leaves

Direction

1. In a medium bowl, stir together the chickpeas, celery, shallot, apple, tahini, lemon juice, honey, mustard, and salt. If needed, add some water to thin the mixture.
2. Place the romaine lettuce leaves on a plate. Fill each with the chickpea filling, using it all. Wrap the leaves around the filling. Serve immediately.

Per Serving

Calories: 397 | fat: 15.1g | protein: 15.1g | carbs: 53.1g | fiber: 15.3g | sodium: 409mg

Turkish Eggplant and Tomatoes Pide with Mint

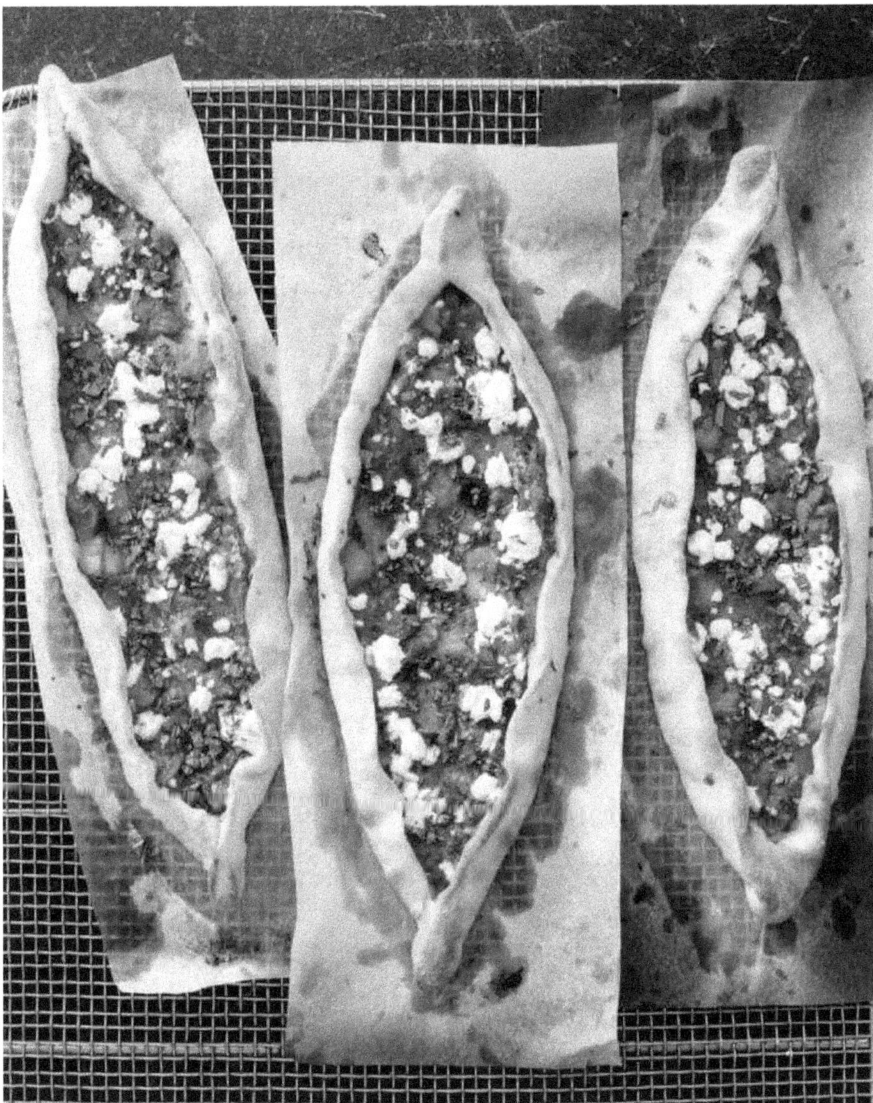

Prep time:

1 day 40 minutes | Cook time: 20 minutes | Makes 6 pides

Ingredients

Dough:

3 cups almond flour

2 teaspoons raw honey

½ teaspoon instant or rapid-rise yeast

1⅓ cups ice water

1 tablespoon extra-virgin olive oil

1½ teaspoons sea salt

Eggplant and Tomato Toppings:

28 ounces (794 g) whole tomatoes, peeled and puréed

5 tablespoons extra-virgin olive oil, divided

1 pound (454 g) eggplant, cut into ½-inch pieces

½ red bell pepper, chopped

Sea salt and ground black pepper, to taste

3 garlic cloves, minced

¼ teaspoon red pepper flakes

½ teaspoon smoked paprika

6 tablespoons minced fresh mint, divided

1½ cups crumbled feta cheese

Direction

Make the Dough

1. Combine the flour, yeast, and honey in a food processor, pulse to combine well. Gently add water while pulsing. Let the dough sit for 10 minutes.
2. Mix the olive oil and salt in the dough and knead the dough until smooth. Wrap in plastic and refrigerate for at least 1 day.

Make the Toppings

3. Heat 2 tablespoons of olive oil in a nonstick skillet over medium-high heat until shimmering.
4. Add the bell pepper, eggplant, and ½ teaspoon of salt. Sauté for 6 minutes or until the eggplant is lightly browned.
5. Add the red pepper flakes, paprika, and garlic. Sauté for 1 minute or until fragrant.
6. Pour in the puréed tomatoes. Bring to a simmer, then cook for 10 minutes or until the mixture is thickened into about 3½ cups.
7. Turn off the heat and mix in 4 tablespoons of mint, salt, and ground black pepper. Set them aside until ready to use.

Make the Turkish Pide

8. Preheat the oven to 500ºF (260ºC). Line three baking sheets with parchment papers.
9. On a clean work surface, divide and shape the dough into six 14 by 5-inch ovals. Transfer the dough to the baking sheets.
10. Brush them with 3 tablespoons of olive oil and spread the eggplant mixture and feta cheese on top.
11. Bake in the preheated oven for 12 minutes or until golden brown. Rotate the pide halfway through the baking time.
12. Remove the pide from the oven and spread with remaining mint and serve immediately.

Per Serving (1 pide)

Calories: 500 | fat: 22.1g | protein: 8.0g | carbs: 69.7g | fiber: 5.8g | sodium: 1001mg

Veg Mix and Blackeye Pea Burritos

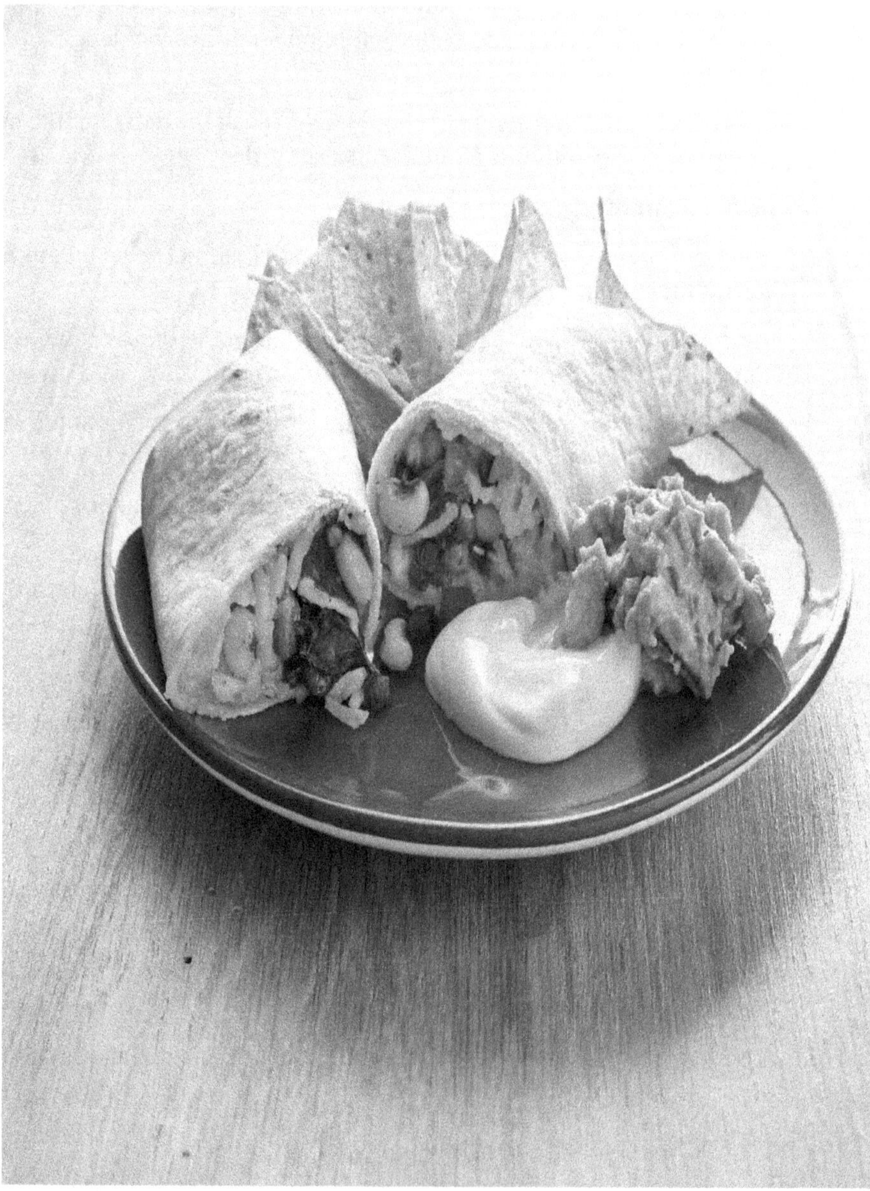

Prep time:

15 minutes | Cook time: 40 minutes | Makes 6 burritos

Ingredients

1 teaspoon olive oil

1 red onion, diced

2 garlic cloves, minced

1 zucchini, chopped

1 tomato, diced

1 bell pepper, any color, deseeded and diced

1 (14-ounce / 397-g) can blackeye peas

2 teaspoons chili powder

Sea salt, to taste

6 whole-grain tortillas

Direction

1. Preheat the oven to 325ºF (160ºC).
2. Heat the olive oil in a nonstick skillet over medium heat or until shimmering.
3. Add the onion and sauté for 5 minutes or until translucent.
4. Add the garlic and sauté for 30 seconds or until fragrant.
5. Add the zucchini and sauté for 5 minutes or until tender.
6. Add the tomato and bell pepper and sauté for 2 minutes or until soft.
7. Fold in the black peas and sprinkle them with chili powder and salt. Stir to mix well.
8. Place the tortillas on a clean work surface, then top them with sautéed vegetables mix.
9. Fold one ends of tortillas over the vegetable mix, then tuck and roll them into burritos.
10. Arrange the burritos in a baking dish, seam side down, then pour the juice remains in the skillet over the burritos.
11. Bake in the preheated oven for 25 minutes or until golden brown.
12. Serve immediately.

Per Serving

Calories: 335 | fat: 16.2g | protein: 12.1g | carbs: 8.3g | fiber: 8.0g | sodium: 214mg

Tuna and Olive Salad Sandwiches

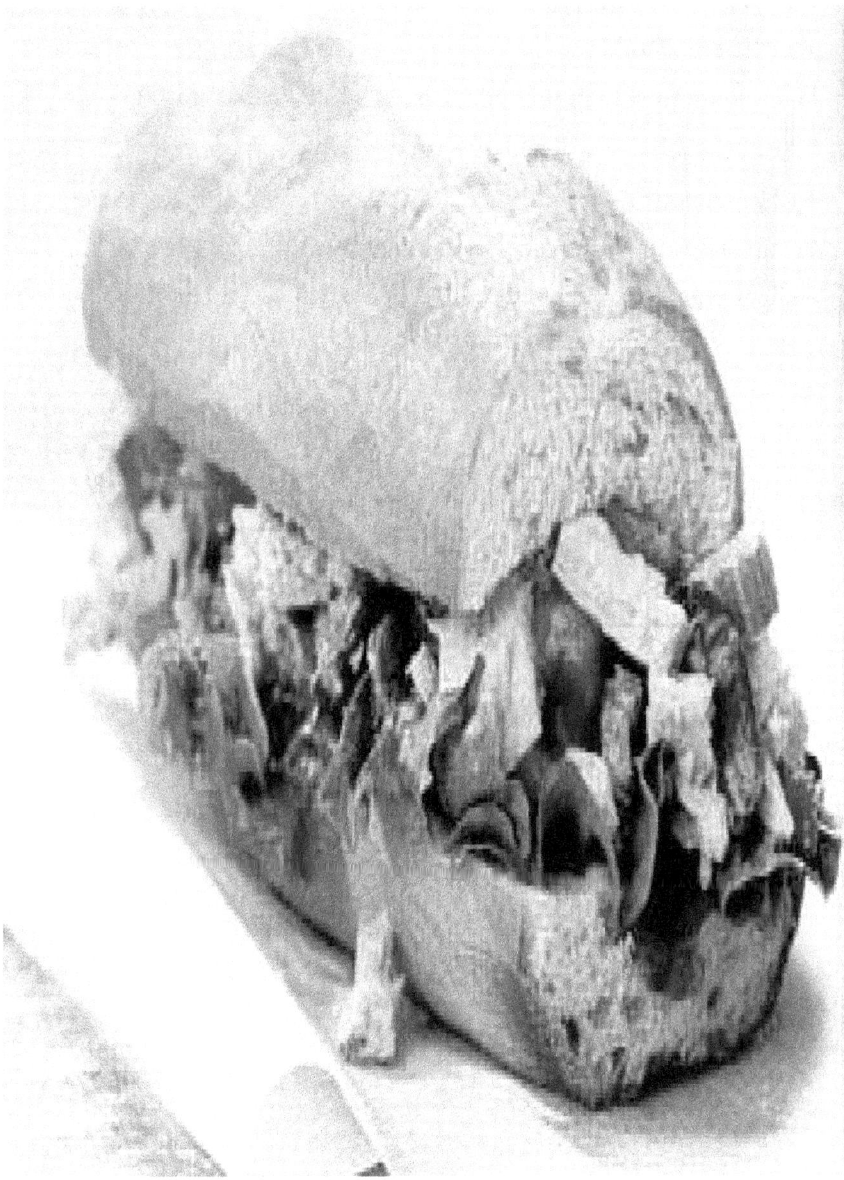

Prep time:

10 minutes | Cook time: 0 minutes | Serves 4

Ingredients

3 tablespoons freshly squeezed lemon juice

2 tablespoons extra-virgin olive oil

1 garlic clove, minced

½ teaspoon freshly ground black pepper

2 (5-ounce / 142-g) cans tuna, drained

1 (2.25-ounce / 64-g) can sliced olives, any green or black variety

½ cup chopped fresh fennel, including fronds

8 slices whole-grain crusty bread

Direction

1. In a medium bowl, whisk together the lemon juice, oil, garlic, and pepper. Add the tuna, olives and fennel to the bowl. Using a fork, separate the tuna into chunks and stir to incorporate all the Ingredients.
2. Divide the tuna salad equally among 4 slices of bread. Top each with the remaining bread slices.
3. Let the sandwiches sit for at least 5 minutes so the zesty filling can soak into the bread before serving.

Per Serving

Calories: 952 | fat: 17.0g | protein: 165.0g | carbs: 37.0g | fiber: 7.0g | sodium: 2572mg

Open-Faced Margherita Sandwiches

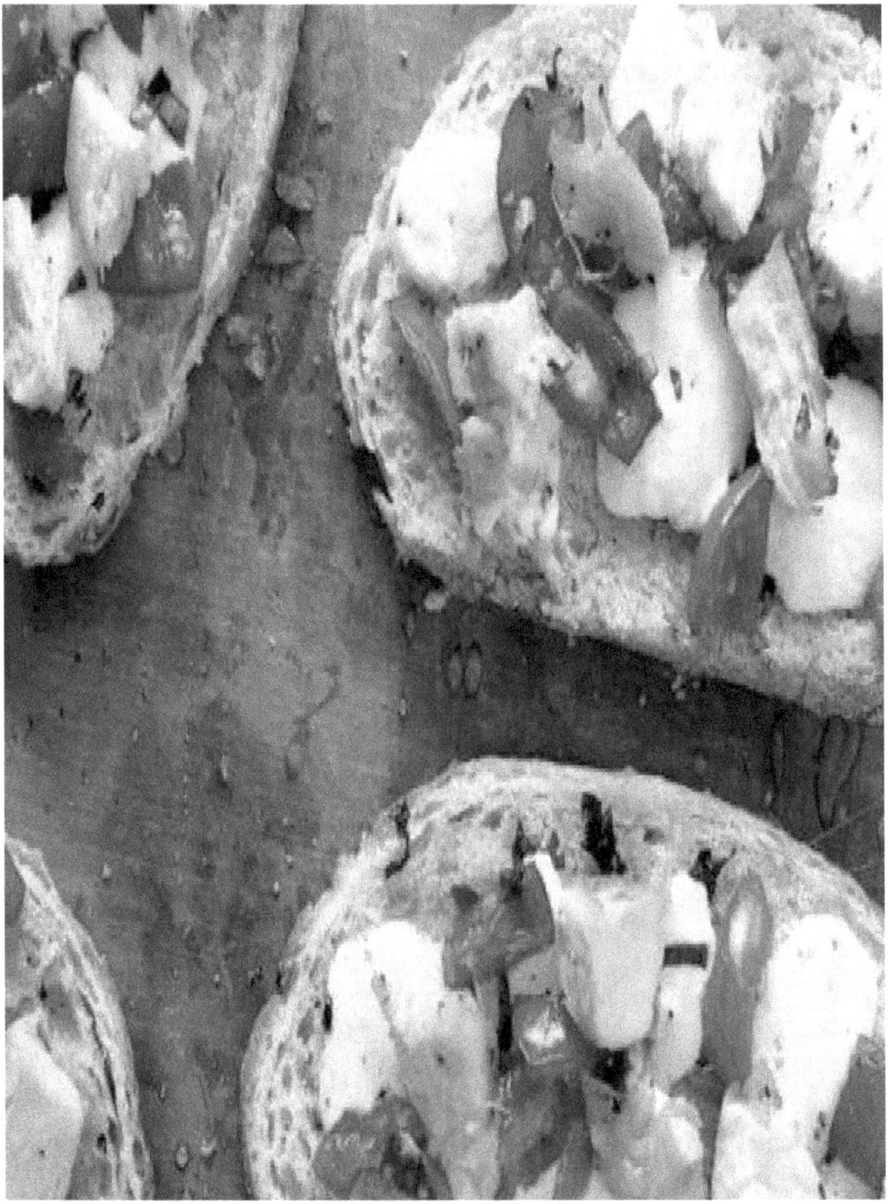

Prep time:

10 minutes | Cook time: 5 minutes | Serves 4

Ingredients

2 (6- to 7-inch) whole-wheat submarine or hoagie rolls, sliced open horizontally

1 tablespoon extra-virgin olive oil

1 garlic clove, halved

1 large ripe tomato, cut into 8 slices

¼ teaspoon dried oregano

1 cup fresh Mozzarella, sliced

¼ cup lightly packed fresh basil leaves, torn into small pieces

¼ teaspoon freshly ground black pepper

Direction

1. Preheat the broiler to High with the rack 4 inches under the heating element.
2. Put the sliced bread on a large, rimmed baking sheet and broil for 1 minute, or until the bread is just lightly toasted. Remove from the oven.
3. Brush each piece of the toasted bread with the oil, and rub a garlic half over each piece.
4. Put the toasted bread back on the baking sheet. Evenly divide the tomato slices on each piece. Sprinkle with the oregano and top with the cheese.
5. Place the baking sheet under the broiler. Set the timer for 1½ minutes, but check after 1 minute. When the cheese is melted and the edges are just starting to get dark brown, remove the sandwiches from the oven.
6. Top each sandwich with the fresh basil and pepper before serving.

Per Serving

Calories: 93 | fat: 2.0g | protein: 10.0g | carbs: 8.0g | fiber: 2.0g | sodium: 313mg

Roasted Vegetable Panini

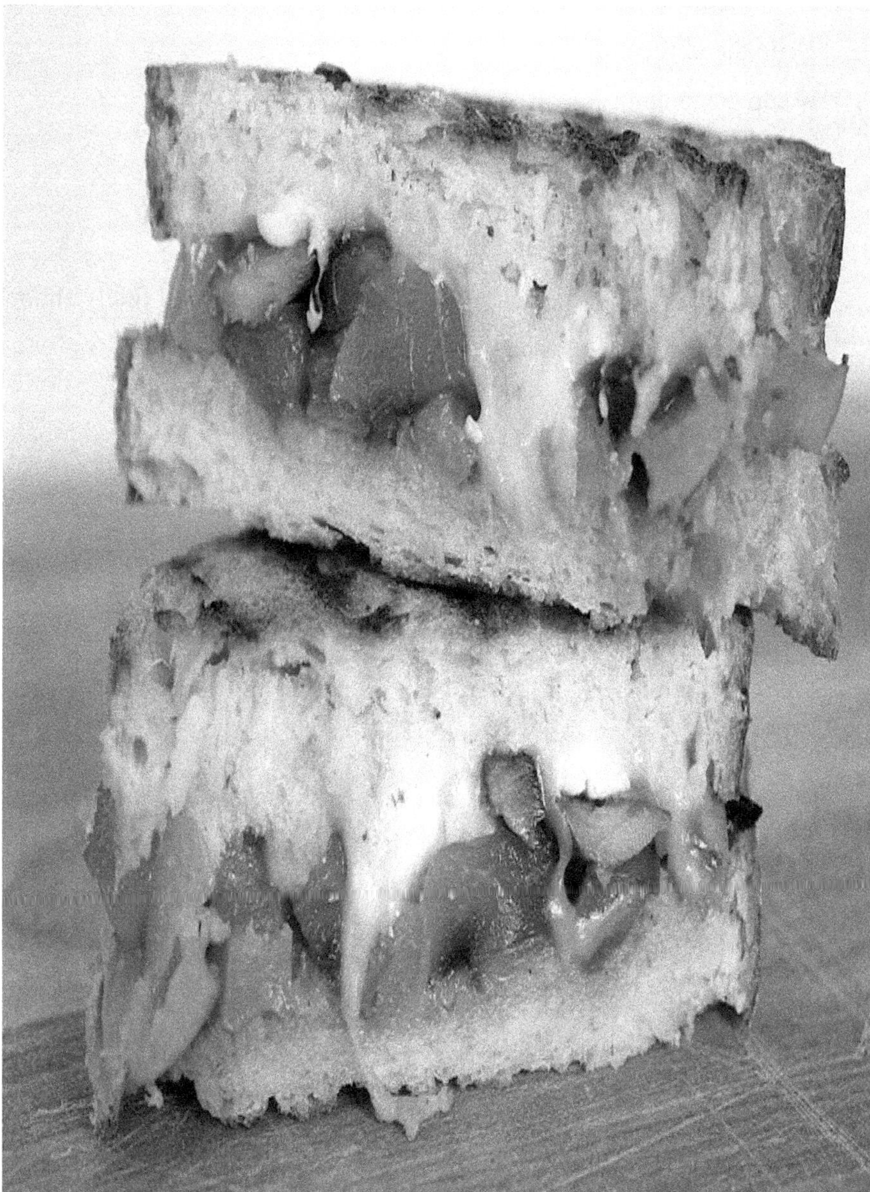

Prep time:

10 minutes | Cook time: 15 minutes | Serves 4

Ingredients

2 tablespoons extra-virgin olive oil, divided

1½ cups diced broccoli

1 cup diced zucchini

¼ cup diced onion

¼ teaspoon dried oregano

⅛ teaspoon kosher or sea salt

⅛ teaspoon freshly ground black pepper

1 (12-ounce / 340-g) jar roasted red peppers, drained and finely chopped

2 tablespoons grated Parmesan or Asiago cheese

1 cup fresh Mozzarella (about 4 ounces / 113 g), sliced

1 (2-foot-long) whole-grain Italian loaf, cut into

4 equal lengths Cooking spray

Direction

1. Place a large, rimmed baking sheet in the oven. Preheat the oven to 450°F (235°C) with the baking sheet inside.
2. In a large bowl, stir together 1 tablespoon of the oil, broccoli, zucchini, onion, oregano, salt and pepper.
3. Remove the baking sheet from the oven and spritz the baking sheet with cooking spray. Spread the vegetable mixture on the baking sheet and roast for 5 minutes, stirring once halfway through cooking.
4. Remove the baking sheet from the oven. Stir in the red peppers and Parmesan cheese.
5. In a large skillet over medium-high heat, heat the remaining 1 tablespoon of the oil.
6. Cut open each section of bread horizontally, but don't cut all the way through. Fill each with the vegetable mix (about ½ cup), and layer 1 ounce (28 g) of sliced Mozzarella cheese on top. Close the sandwiches, and place two of them on the skillet. Place a heavy object on top and grill for 2½ minutes. Flip the sandwiches and grill for another 2½ minutes.
7. Repeat the grilling process with the remaining two sandwiches.
8. Serve hot.

Per Serving

Calories: 116 | fat: 4.0g | protein: 12.0g | carbs: 9.0g | fiber: 3.0g | sodium: 569mg

White Pizzas with Arugula and Spinach

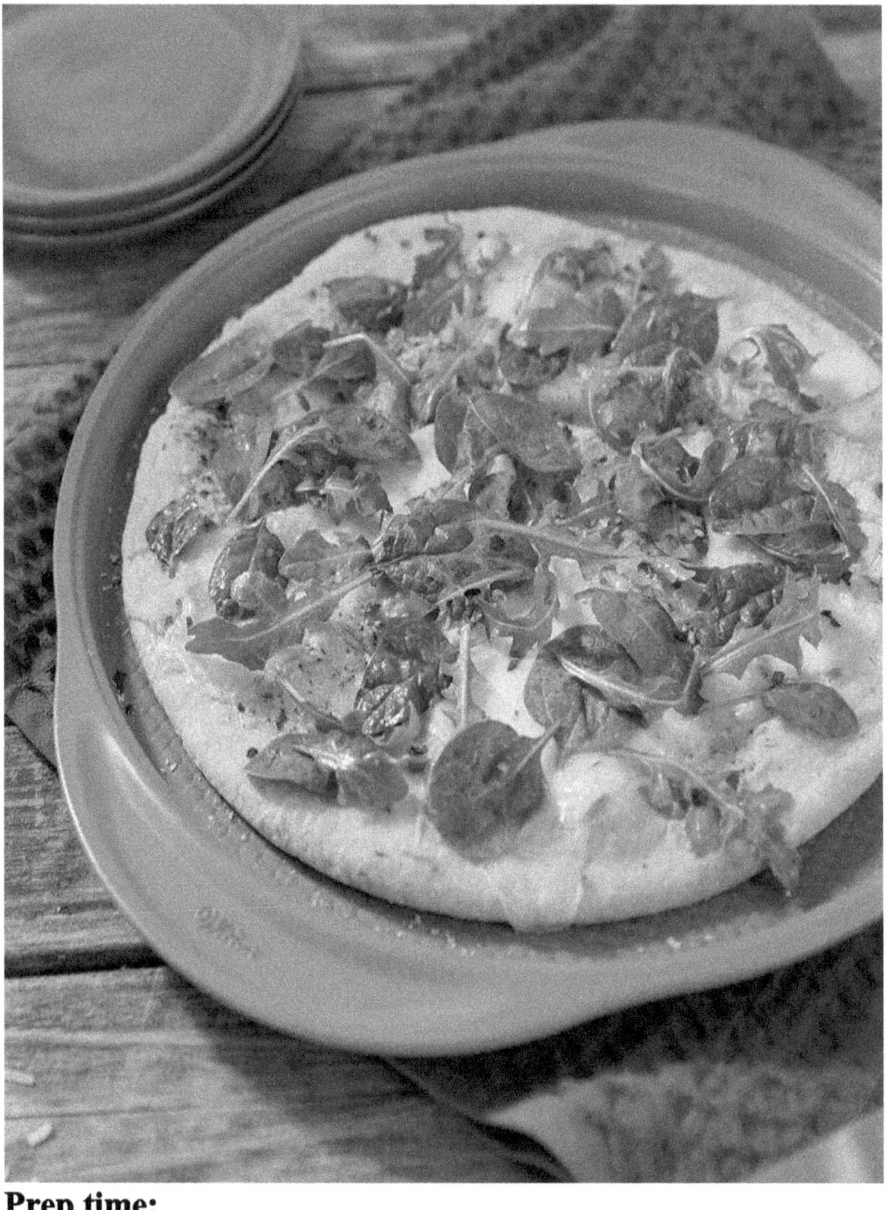

Prep time:

10 minutes | Cook time: 20 minutes | Serves 4

Ingredients

1 pound (454 g) refrigerated fresh pizza dough

2 tablespoons extra-virgin olive oil, divided

½ cup thinly sliced onion

2 garlic cloves, minced

3 cups baby spinach

3 cups arugula

1 tablespoon water

¼ teaspoon freshly ground black pepper

1 tablespoon freshly squeezed lemon juice

½ cup shredded Parmesan cheese

½ cup crumbled goat cheese

Cooking spray

Direction

1. Preheat the oven to 500°F (260°C). Spritz a large, rimmed baking sheet with cooking spray.
2. Take the pizza dough out of the refrigerator.
3. Heat 1 tablespoon of the oil in a large skillet over medium heat. Add the onion to the skillet and cook for 4 minutes, stirring constantly. Add the garlic and cook for 1 minute, stirring constantly.
4. Stir in the spinach, arugula, water and pepper. Cook for about 2 minutes, stirring constantly, or until all the greens are coated with oil and they start to cook down. Remove the skillet from the heat and drizzle with the lemon juice.
5. On a lightly floured work surface, form the pizza dough into a 12-inch circle or a 10-by-12-inch rectangle, using a rolling pin or by stretching with your hands.
6. Place the dough on the prepared baking sheet. Brush the dough with the remaining 1 tablespoon of the oil. Spread the cooked greens on top of the dough to within ½ inch of the edge. Top with the Parmesan cheese and goat cheese.
7. Bake in the preheated oven for 10 to 12 minutes, or until the crust starts to brown around the edges.
8. Remove from the oven and transfer the pizza to a cutting board. Cut into eight pieces before serving.

Per Serving

Calories: 521 | fat: 31.0g | protein: 23.0g | carbs: 38.0g | fiber: 4.0g | sodium: 1073mg

Za'atar Pizza

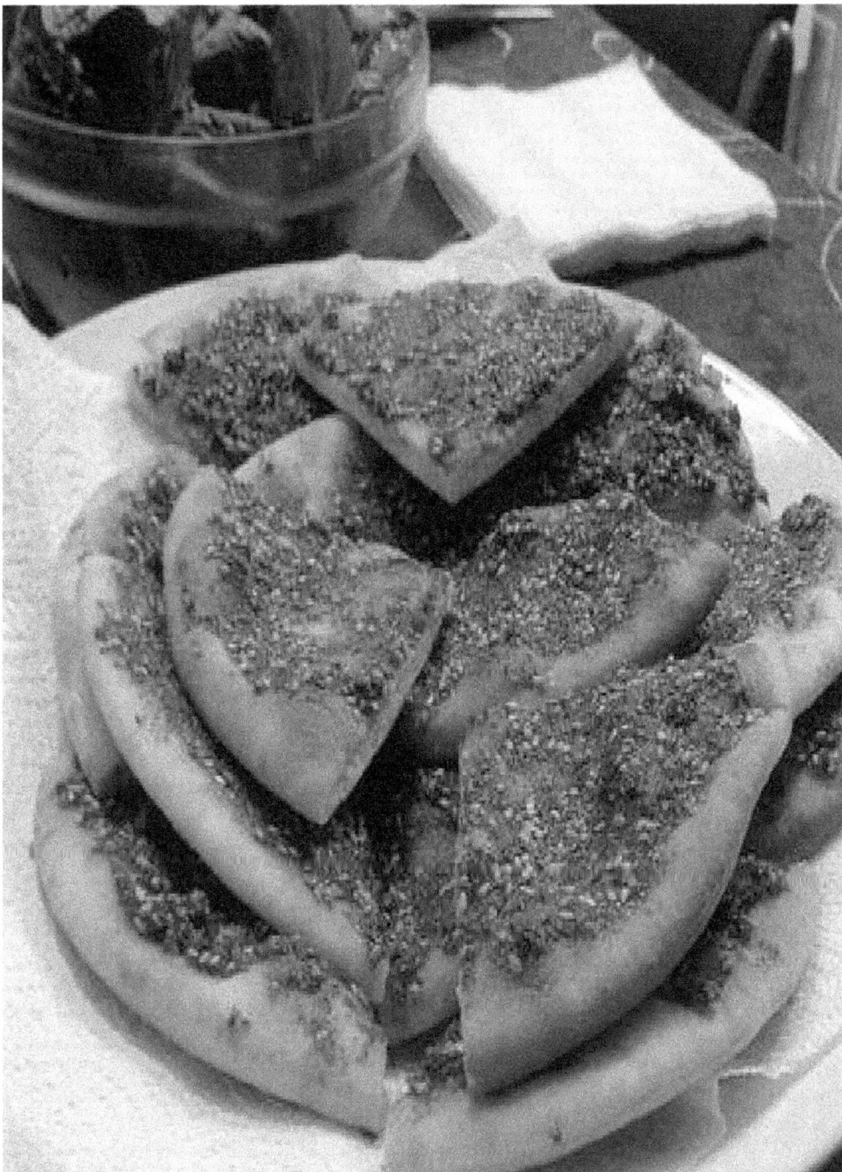

Prep time:

10 minutes | Cook time: 1o to 12 minutes | Serves 4 to 6

Ingredients

1 sheet puff pastry

¼ cup extra-virgin olive oil

⅓ cup za'atar seasoning

Direction

1. Preheat the oven to 350°F (180°C). Line a baking sheet with parchment paper.
2. Place the puff pastry on the prepared baking sheet. Cut the pastry into desired slices.
3. Brush the pastry with the olive oil. Sprinkle with the za'atar seasoning.
4. Put the pastry in the oven and bake for 10 to 12 minutes, or until edges are lightly browned and puffed up.
5. Serve warm.

Per Serving

Calories: 374 | fat: 30.0g | protein: 3.0g | carbs: 20.0g | fiber: 1.0g | sodium: 166mg

Zucchini Hummus Wraps

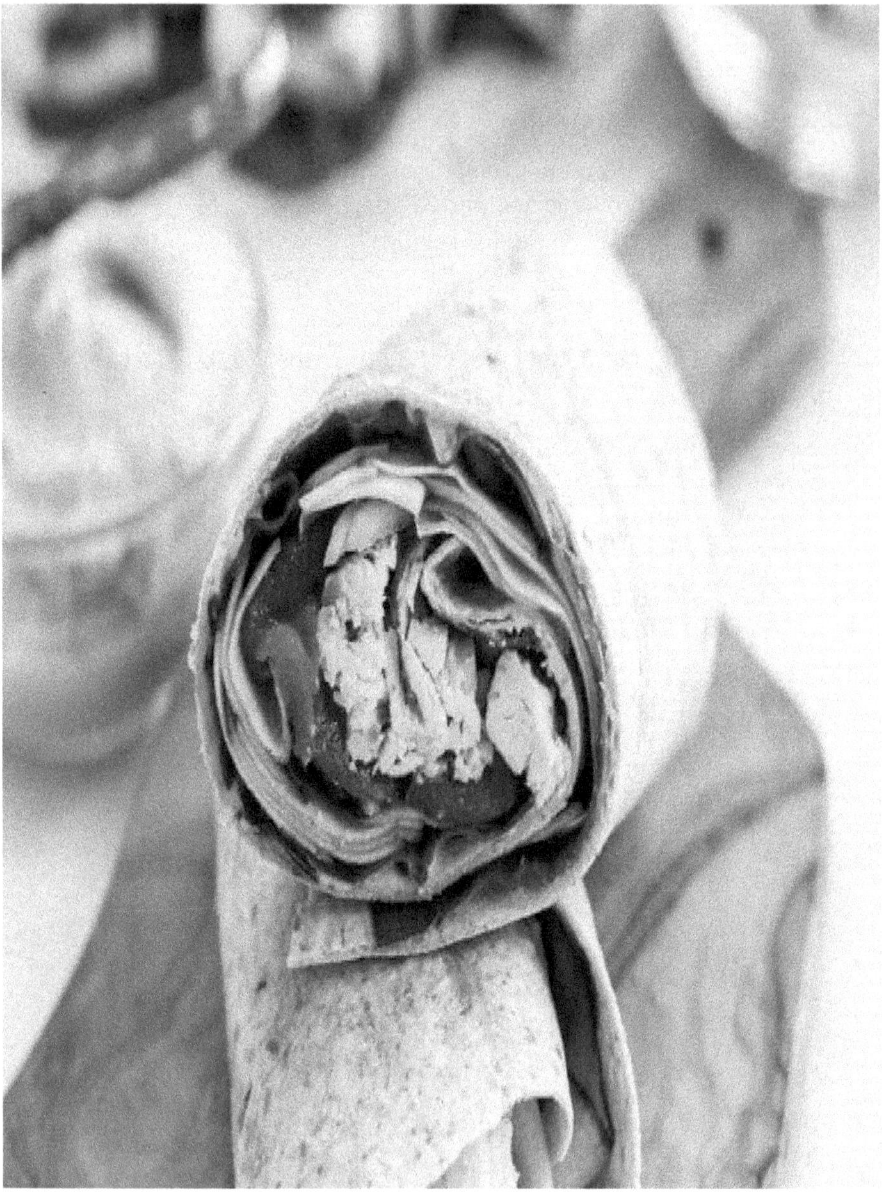

Prep time:

15 minutes | Cook time: 6 minutes | Serves 2

Ingredients

1 zucchini, ends removed, thinly sliced lengthwise

½ teaspoon dried oregano

¼ teaspoon freshly ground black pepper

¼ teaspoon garlic powder

¼ cup hummus

2 whole wheat tortillas

2 Roma tomatoes, cut lengthwise into slices

1 cup chopped kale

2 tablespoons chopped red onion

½ teaspoon ground cumin

Direction

1. In a skillet over medium heat, add the zucchini slices and cook for 3 minutes per side. Sprinkle with the oregano, pepper, and garlic powder and remove from the heat.
2. Spread 2 tablespoons of hummus on each tortilla. Lay half the zucchini in the center of each tortilla. Top with tomato slices, kale, red onion, and ¼ teaspoon of cumin. Wrap tightly and serve.

Per Serving

Calories: 248 | fat: 8.1g | protein: 9.1g | carbs: 37.1g | fiber: 8.1g | sodium: m

Baked Rolled Oat with Pears and Pecans

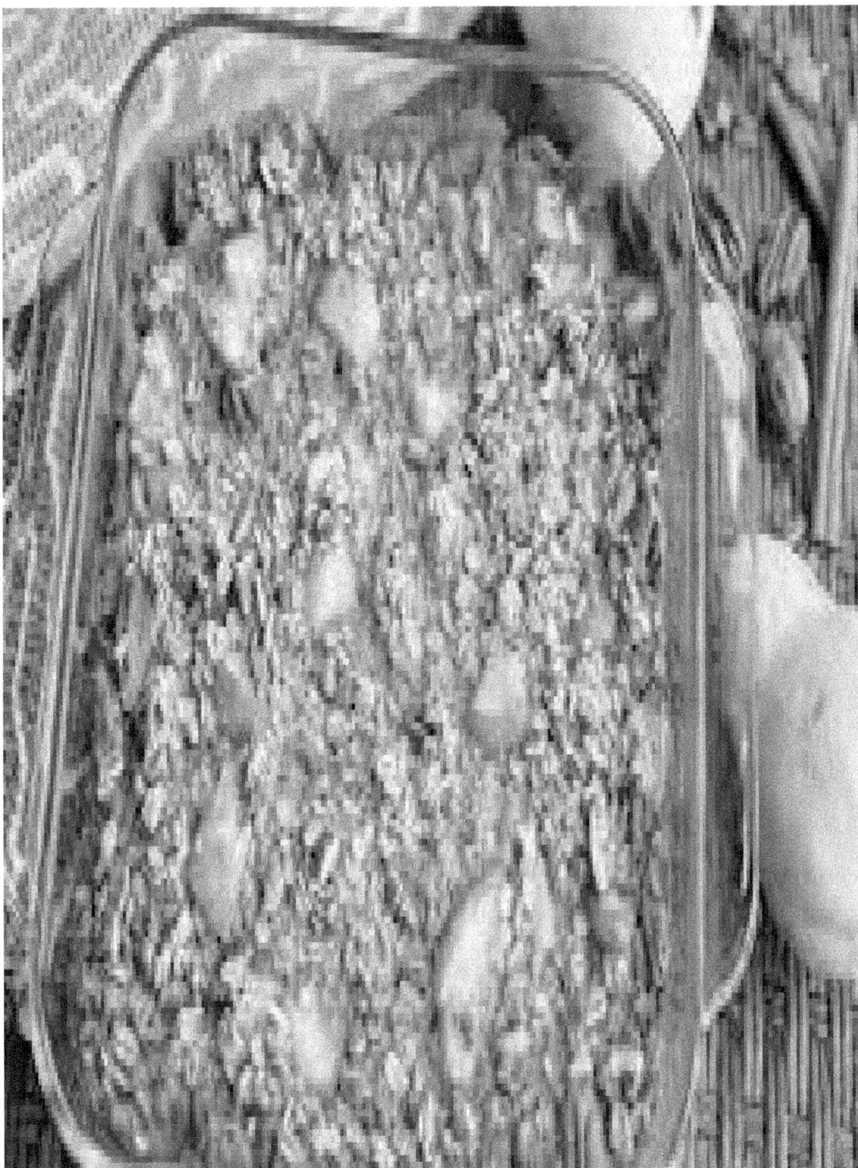

Prep time:

15 minutes | Cook time: 30 minutes | Serves 6

Ingredients

2 tablespoons coconut oil, melted, plus more for greasing the pan

3 ripe pears, cored and diced

2 cups unsweetened almond milk

1 tablespoon pure vanilla extract

¼ cup pure maple syrup

2 cups gluten-free rolled oats

½ cup raisins

¾ cup chopped pecans

¼ teaspoon ground nutmeg

1 teaspoon ground cinnamon

½ teaspoon ground ginger

¼ teaspoon sea salt

Direction

1. Preheat the oven to 350ºF (180ºC). Grease a baking dish with melted coconut oil, then spread the pears in a single layer on the baking dish evenly.
2. Combine the almond milk, vanilla extract, maple syrup, and coconut oil in a bowl. Stir to mix well.
3. Combine the remaining **Ingredients** in a separate large bowl. Stir to mix well. Fold the almond milk mixture in the bowl, then pour the mixture over the pears.
4. Place the baking dish in the preheated oven and bake for 30 minutes or until lightly browned and set.
5. Serve immediately.

Per Serving

Calories: 479 | fat: 34.9g | protein: 8.8g | carbs: 50.1g | fiber: 10.8g | sodium: 113mg

Brown Rice Pilaf with Pistachios and Raisins

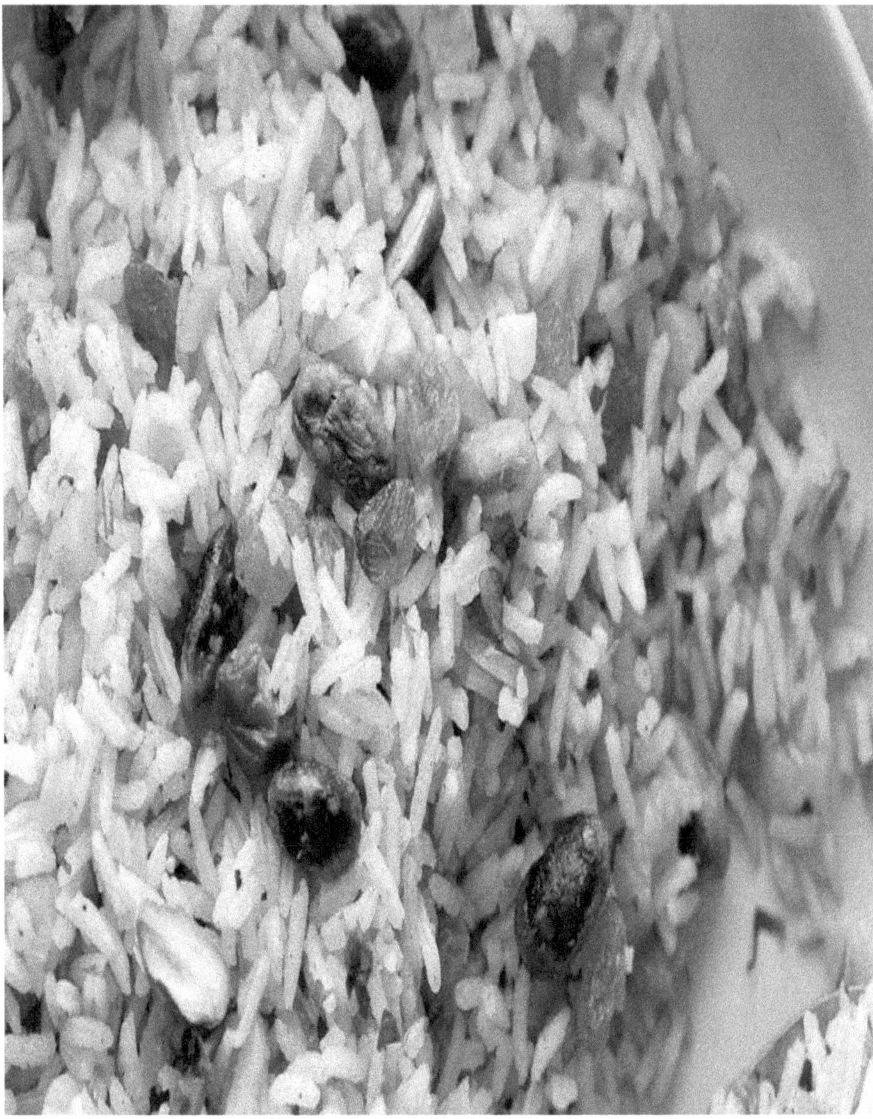

Prep time:

5 minutes | Cook time: 15 minutes | Serves 6

Ingredients

1 tablespoon extra-virgin olive oil

1 cup chopped onion

½ cup shredded carrot

½ teaspoon ground cinnamon

1 teaspoon ground cumin

2 cups brown rice

1¾ cups pure orange juice

¼ cup water

½ cup shelled pistachios

1 cup golden raisins

½ cup chopped fresh chives

Direction

1. Heat the olive oil in a saucepan over medium-high heat until shimmering.
2. Add the onion and sauté for 5 minutes or until translucent.
3. Add the carrots, cinnamon, and cumin, then sauté for 1 minutes or until aromatic.
4. Pour int the brown rice, orange juice, and water. Bring to a boil. Reduce the heat to medium-low and simmer for 7 minutes or until the liquid is almost absorbed.
5. Transfer the rice mixture in a large serving bowl, then spread with pistachios, raisins, and chives. Serve immediately.

Per Serving

Calories: 264 | fat: 7.1g | protein: 5.2g | carbs: 48.9g | fiber: 4.0g | sodium: 86mg

Cherry, Apricot, and Pecan Brown Rice Bowl

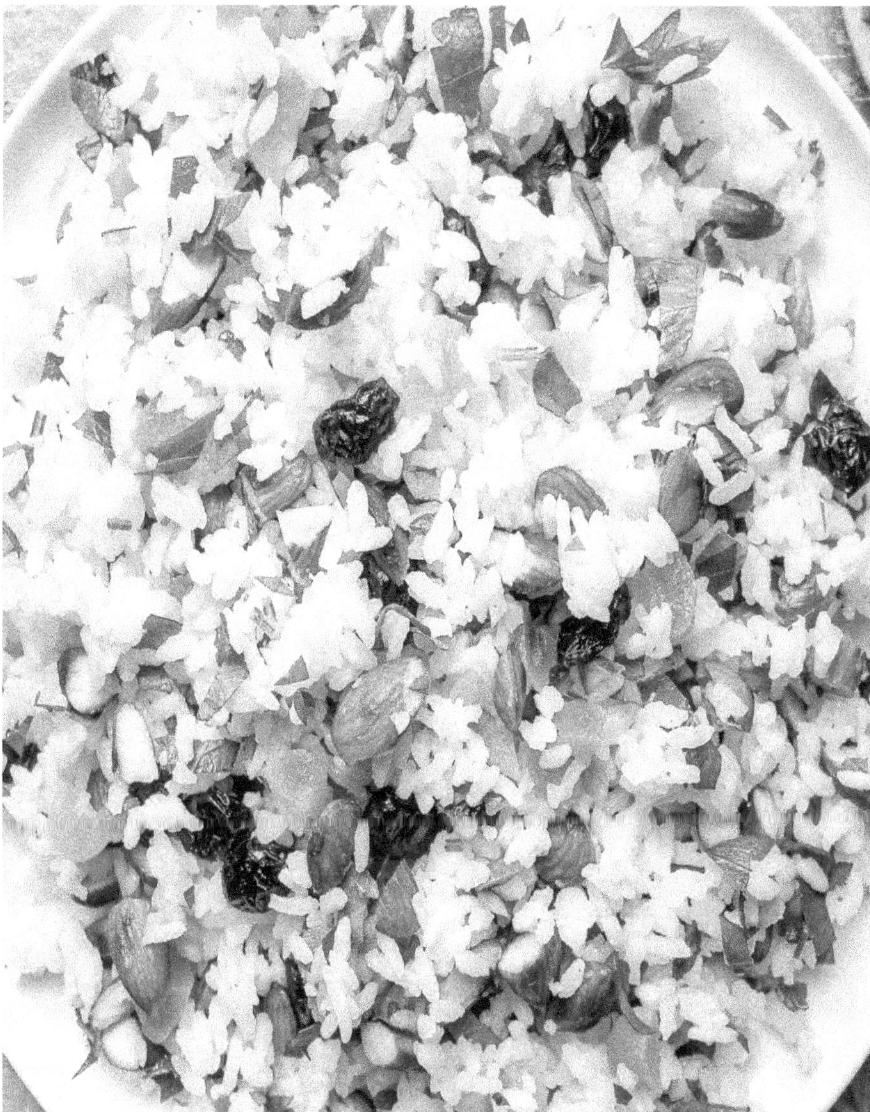

Prep time:

15 minutes | Cook time: 1 hour 1 minutes | Serves 2

Ingredients

2 tablespoons olive oil

2 green onions, sliced

½ cup brown rice

1 cup low -sodium chicken stock

2 tablespoons dried cherries

4 dried apricots, chopped

2 tablespoons pecans, toasted and chopped

Sea salt and freshly ground pepper, to taste

Direction

1. Heat the olive oil in a medium saucepan over medium-high heat until shimmering.
2. Add the green onions and sauté for 1 minutes or until fragrant.
3. Add the rice. Stir to mix well, then pour in the chicken stock.
4. Bring to a boil. Reduce the heat to low. Cover and simmer for 50 minutes or until the brown rice is soft.
5. Add the cherries, apricots, and pecans, and simmer for 10 more minutes or until the fruits are tender.
6. Pour them in a large serving bowl. Fluff with a fork. Sprinkle with sea salt and freshly ground pepper. Serve immediately.

Per Serving

Calories: 451 | fat: 25.9g | protein: 8.2g | carbs: 50.4g | fiber: 4.6g | sodium: 122mg

Curry Apple Couscous with Leeks and Pecans

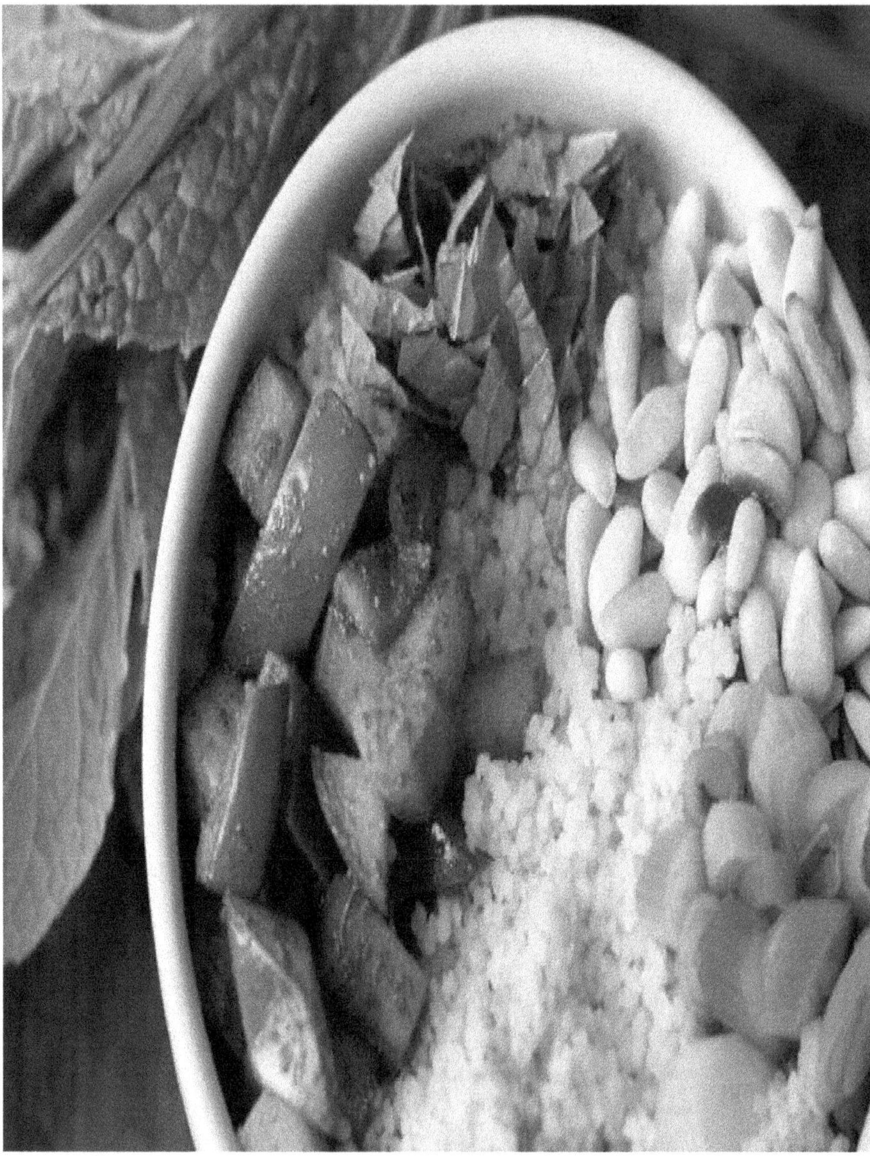

Prep time:

10 minutes | Cook time: 8 minutes | Serves 4

Ingredients

2 teaspoons extra-virgin olive oil

2 leeks, white parts only, sliced

1 apple, diced

2 cups cooked couscous

2 tablespoons curry powder

½ cup chopped pecans

Direction

1. Heat the olive oil in a skillet over medium heat until shimmering.
2. Add the leeks and sauté for 5 minutes or until soft.
3. Add the diced apple and cook for 3 more minutes until tender.
4. Add the couscous and curry powder. Stir to combine.
5. Transfer them in a large serving bowl, then mix in the pecans and serve.

Per Serving

Calories: 254 | fat: 11.9g | protein: 5.4g | carbs: 34.3g | fiber: 5.9g | sodium: 15mg

Lebanese Flavor Broken Thin Noodles

Prep time:

10 minutes | Cook time: 25 minutes | Serves 6

Ingredients

1 tablespoon extra-virgin olive oil

1 (3-ounce / 85-g) cup vermicelli, broken into 1- to 1½-inch pieces

3 cups shredded cabbage

1 cup brown rice

3 cups low-sodium vegetable soup

½ cup water

2 garlic cloves, mashed

¼ teaspoon sea salt

⅛ teaspoon crushed red pepper flakes

½ cup coarsely chopped cilantro

Fresh lemon slices, for serving

Direction

1. Heat the olive oil in a saucepan over medium-high heat until shimmering.
2. Add the vermicelli and sauté for 3 minutes or until toasted.
3. Add the cabbage and sauté for 4 minutes or until tender.
4. Pour in the brown rice, vegetable soup, and water. Add the garlic and sprinkle with salt and red pepper flakes.
5. Bring to a boil over high heat. Reduce the heat to medium low. Put the lid on and simmer for another 10 minutes.
6. Turn off the heat, then let sit for 5 minutes without opening the lid.
7. Pour them on a large serving platter and spread with cilantro. Squeeze the lemon slices over and serve warm.

Per Serving

Calories: 127 | fat: 3.1g | protein: 4.2g | carbs: 22.9g | fiber: 3.0g | sodium: 224mg

Lemony Farro and Avocado Bowl

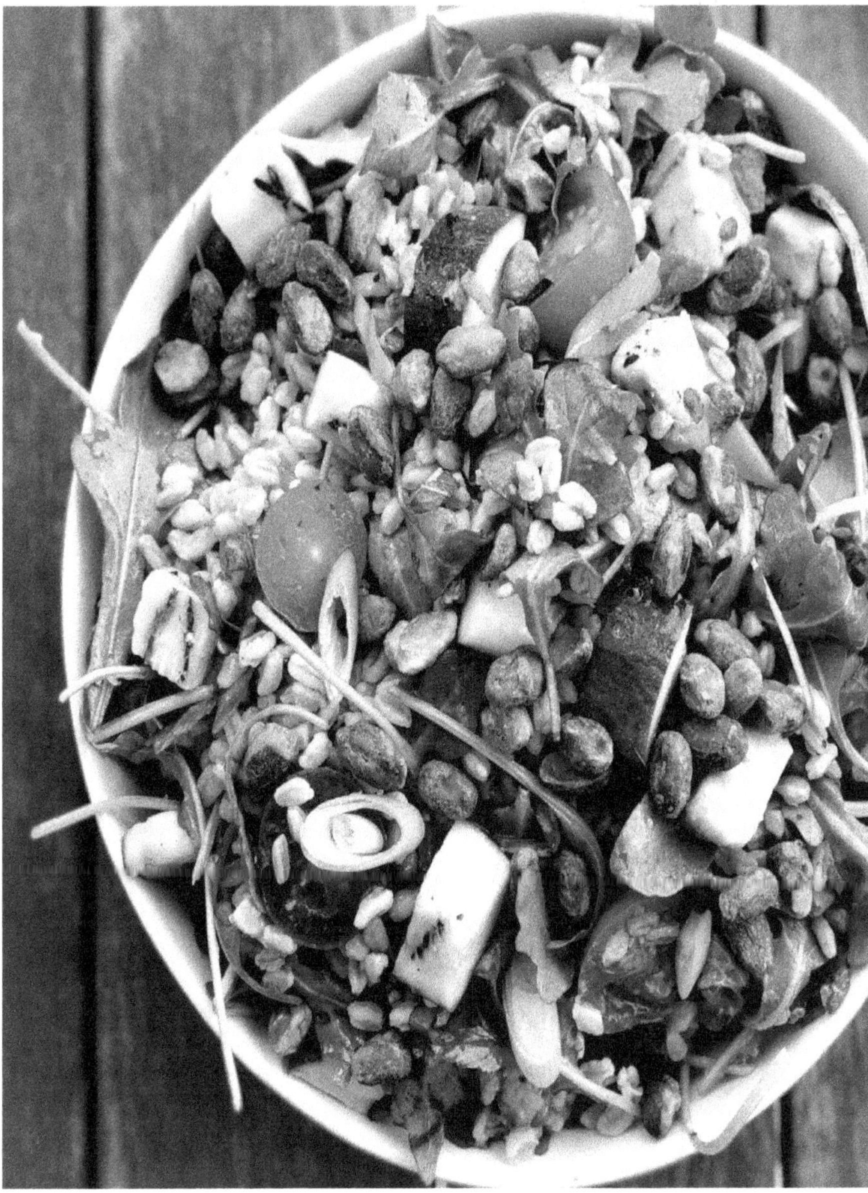

Prep time:

5 minutes | Cook time: 25 minutes | Serves 4

Ingredients

1 tablespoon plus 2 teaspoons extra-virgin olive oil, divided

½ medium onion, chopped

1 carrot, shredded

2 garlic cloves, minced

1 (6-ounce / 170-g) cup pearled farro

2 cups low-sodium vegetable soup

2 avocados, peeled, pitted, and sliced

Zest and juice of 1 small lemon

¼ teaspoon sea salt

Direction

1. Heat 1 tablespoon of olive oil in a saucepan over medium-high heat until shimmering.
2. Add the onion and sauté for 5 minutes or until translucent.
3. Add the carrot and garlic and sauté for 1 minute or until fragrant.
4. Add the farro and pour in the vegetable soup. Bring to a boil over high heat. Reduce the heat to low. Put the lid on and simmer for 20 minutes or until the farro is al dente.
5. Transfer the farro in a large serving bowl, then fold in the avocado slices. Sprinkle with lemon zest and salt, then drizzle with lemon juice and 2 teaspoons of olive oil.
6. Stir to mix well and serve immediately.

Per Serving

Calories: 210 | fat: 11.1g | protein: 4.2g | carbs: 27.9g | fiber: 7.0g | sodium: 152mg

Rice and Blueberry Stuffed Sweet Potatoes

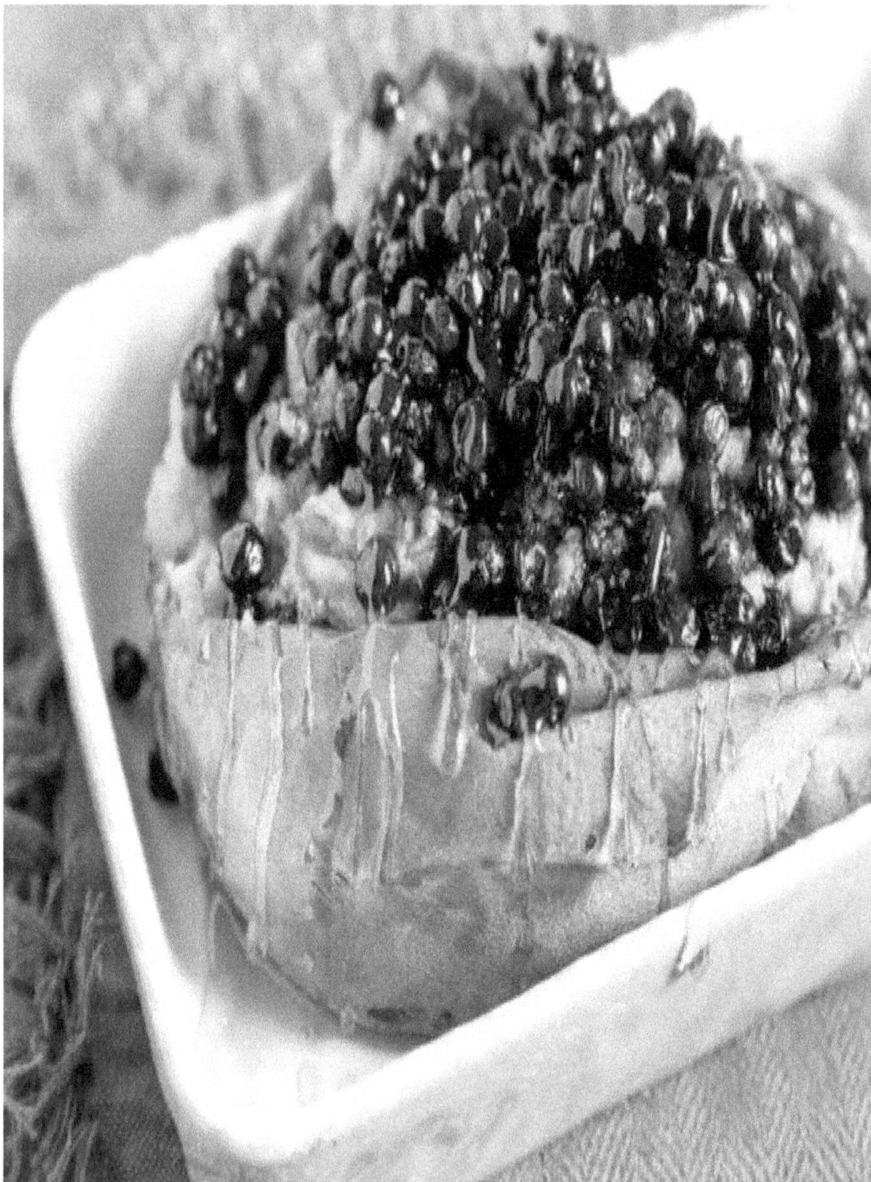

Prep time:

15 minutes | Cook time: 20 minutes | Serves 4

Ingredients

2 cups cooked wild rice

½ cup dried blueberries

½ cup chopped hazelnuts

½ cup shredded Swiss chard

1 teaspoon chopped fresh thyme

1 scallion, white and green parts, peeled and thinly sliced

Sea salt and freshly ground black pepper, to taste

4 sweet potatoes, baked in the skin until tender

Direction

1. Preheat the oven to 400ºF (205ºC).
2. Combine all the **Ingredients,** except for the sweet potatoes, in a large bowl. Stir to mix well.
3. Cut the top third of the sweet potato off length wire, then scoop most of the sweet potato flesh out.
4. Fill the potato with the wild rice mixture, then set the sweet potato on a greased baking sheet.
5. Bake in the preheated oven for 20 minutes or until the sweet potato skin is lightly charred.
6. Serve immediately.

Per Serving

Calories: 393 | fat: 7.1g | protein: 10.2g | carbs: 76.9g | fiber: 10.0g | sodium: 93mg

Slow Cooked Turkey and Brown Rice

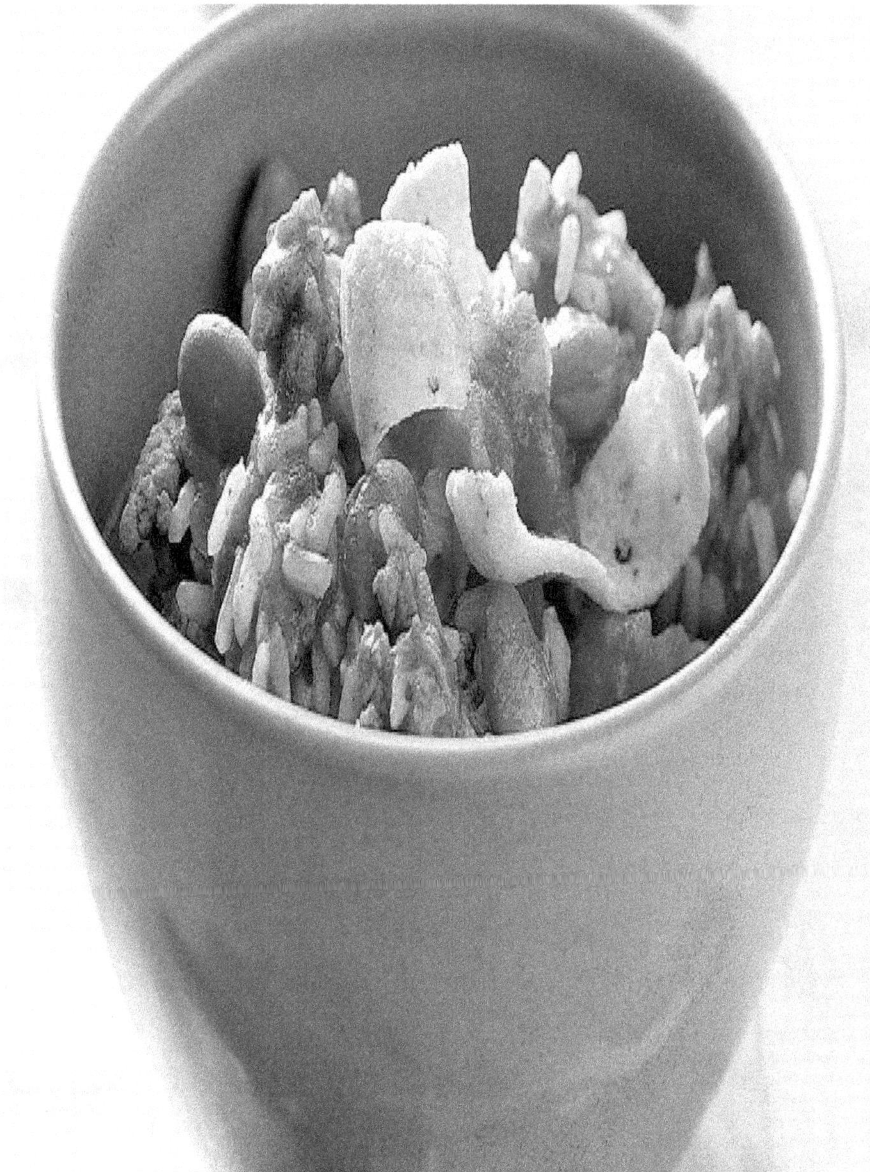

Prep time:

20 minutes | Cook time: 3 hours 10 minutes | Serves 6

Ingredients

1 tablespoon extra-virgin olive oil

1½ pounds (680 g) ground turkey

2 tablespoons chopped fresh sage, divided

2 tablespoons chopped fresh thyme, divided

1 teaspoon sea salt

½ teaspoon ground black pepper

2 cups brown rice

1 (14-ounce / 397-g) can stewed tomatoes, with the juice

¼ cup pitted and sliced Kalamata olives

3 medium zucchini, sliced thinly

¼ cup chopped fresh flat-leaf parsley

1 medium yellow onion, chopped

1 tablespoon plus 1 teaspoon balsamic vinegar

2 cups low-sodium chicken stock

2 garlic cloves, minced

½ cup grated Parmesan cheese, for serving

Direction

1. Heat the olive oil in a nonstick skillet over medium-high heat until shimmering.
2. Add the ground turkey and sprinkle with 1 tablespoon of sage, 1 tablespoon of thyme, salt and ground black pepper.
3. Sauté for 10 minutes or until the ground turkey is lightly browned.
4. Pour them in the slow cooker, then pour in the remaining **Ingredients,** except for the Parmesan. Stir to mix well.
5. Put the lid on and cook on high for 3 hours or until the rice and vegetables are tender.
6. Pour them in a large serving bowl, then spread with Parmesan cheese before serving.

Per Serving

Calories: 499 | fat: 16.4g | protein: 32.4g | carbs: 56.5g | fiber: 4.7g | sodium: 758mg

Papaya, Jicama, and Peas Rice Bowl

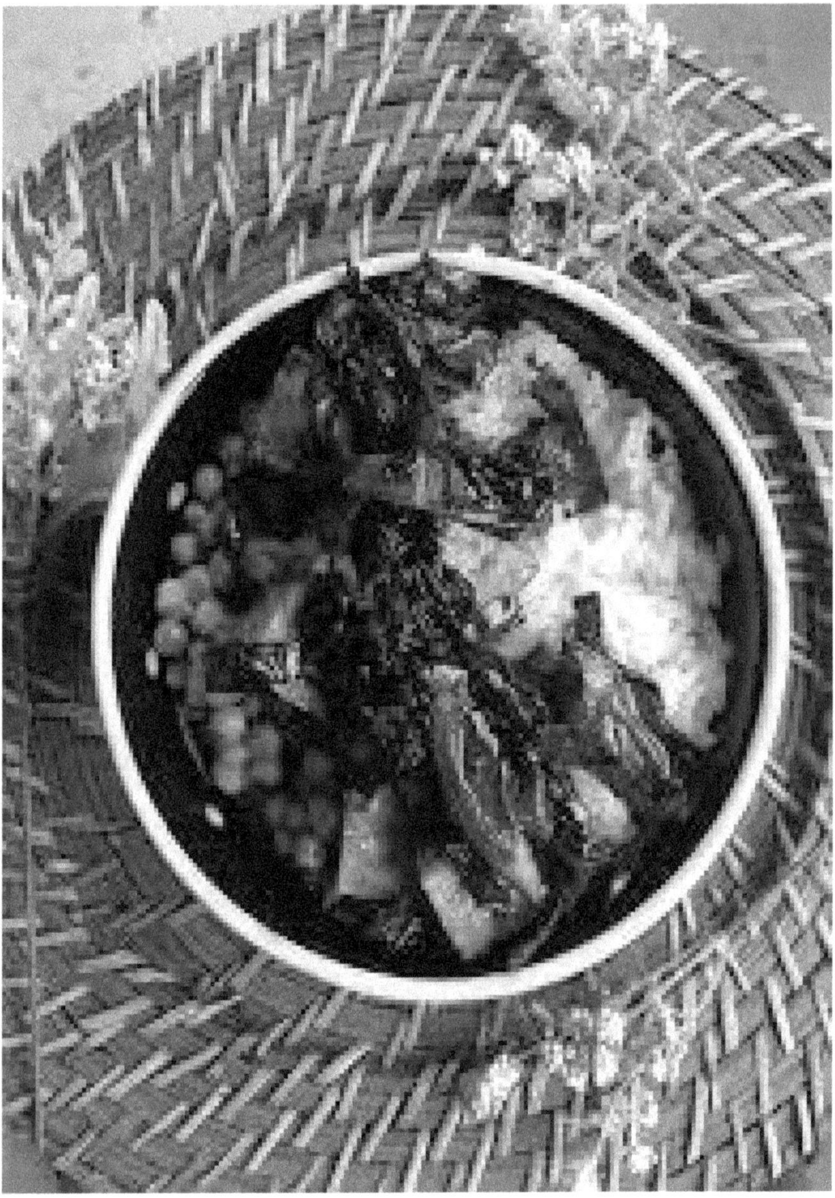

Prep time:

20 minutes | Cook time: 45 minutes | Serves 4

Ingredients

Sauce:

Juice of ¼ lemon

2 teaspoons chopped fresh basil

1 tablespoon raw honey

1 tablespoon extra-virgin olive oil

Sea salt, to taste

Rice:

1½ cups wild rice

2 papayas, peeled, seeded, and diced

1 jicama, peeled and shredded

1 cup snow peas, julienned

2 cups shredded cabbage

1 scallion, white and green parts, chopped

Direction

1. Combine the **Ingredients** for the sauce in a bowl. Stir to mix well. Set aside until ready to use.
2. Pour the wild rice in a saucepan, then pour in enough water to cover. Bring to a boil.
3. Reduce the heat to low, then simmer for 45 minutes or until the wild rice is soft and plump. Drain and transfer to a large serving bowl.
4. Top the rice with papayas, jicama, peas, cabbage, and scallion. Pour the sauce over and stir to mix well before serving.

Per Serving

Calories: 446 | fat: 7.9g | protein: 13.1g | carbs: 85.8g | fiber: 16.0g | sodium: 70mg

Black Bean Chili with Mangoes

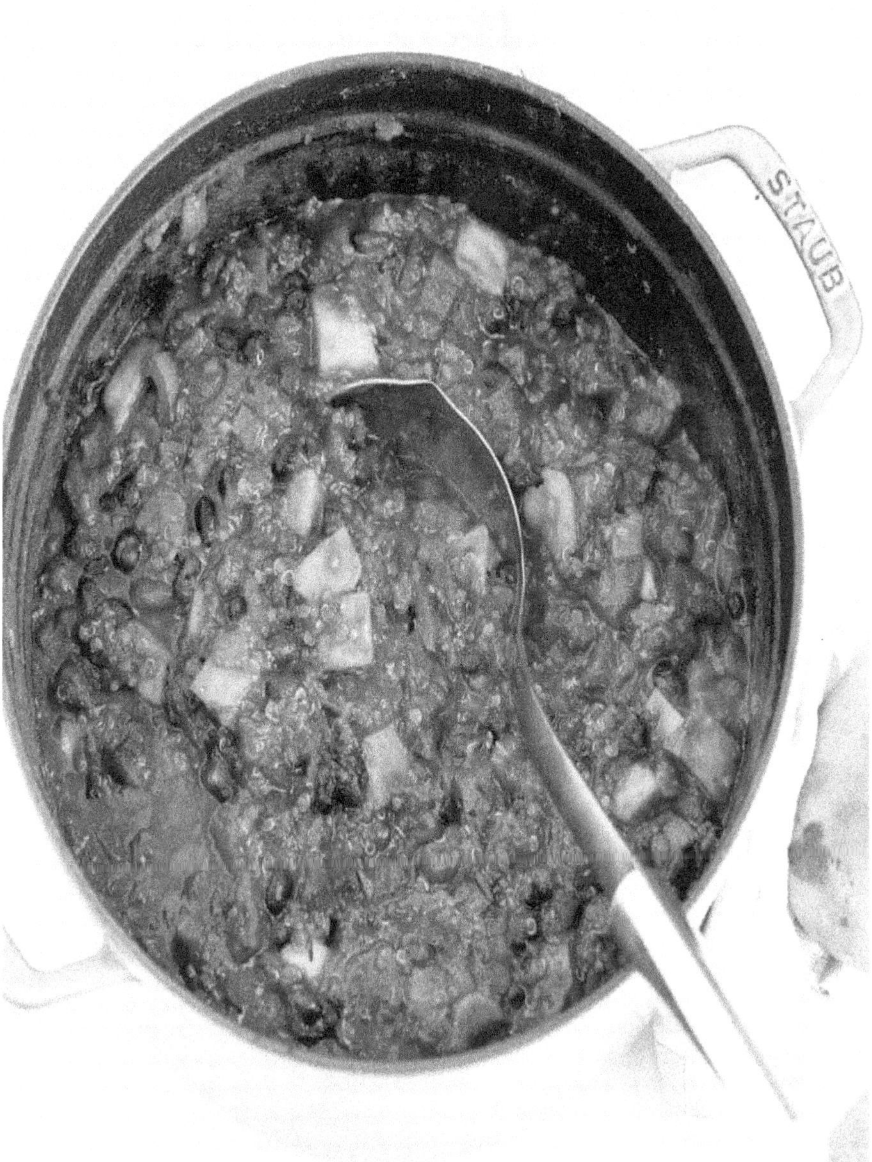

Prep time:

10 minutes | Cook time: 10 minutes | Serves 4

Ingredients

2 tablespoons coconut oil

1 onion, chopped

2 (15-ounce / 425-g) cans black beans, drained and rinsed

1 tablespoon chili powder

1 teaspoon sea salt

¼ teaspoon freshly ground black pepper

1 cup water

2 ripe mangoes, sliced thinly

¼ cup chopped fresh cilantro, divided

¼ cup sliced scallions, divided

Direction

1. Heat the coconut oil in a pot over high heat until melted.
2. Put the onion in the pot and sauté for 5 minutes or until translucent.
3. Add the black beans to the pot. Sprinkle with chili powder, salt, and ground black pepper. Pour in the water. Stir to mix well.
4. Bring to a boil. Reduce the heat to low, then simmering for 5 minutes or until the beans are tender.
5. Turn off the heat and mix in the mangoes, then garnish with scallions and cilantro before serving.

Per Serving

Calories: 430 | fat: 9.1g | protein: 20.2g | carbs: 71.9g | fiber: 22.0g | sodium: 608mg

Israeli Style Eggplant and Chickpea Salad

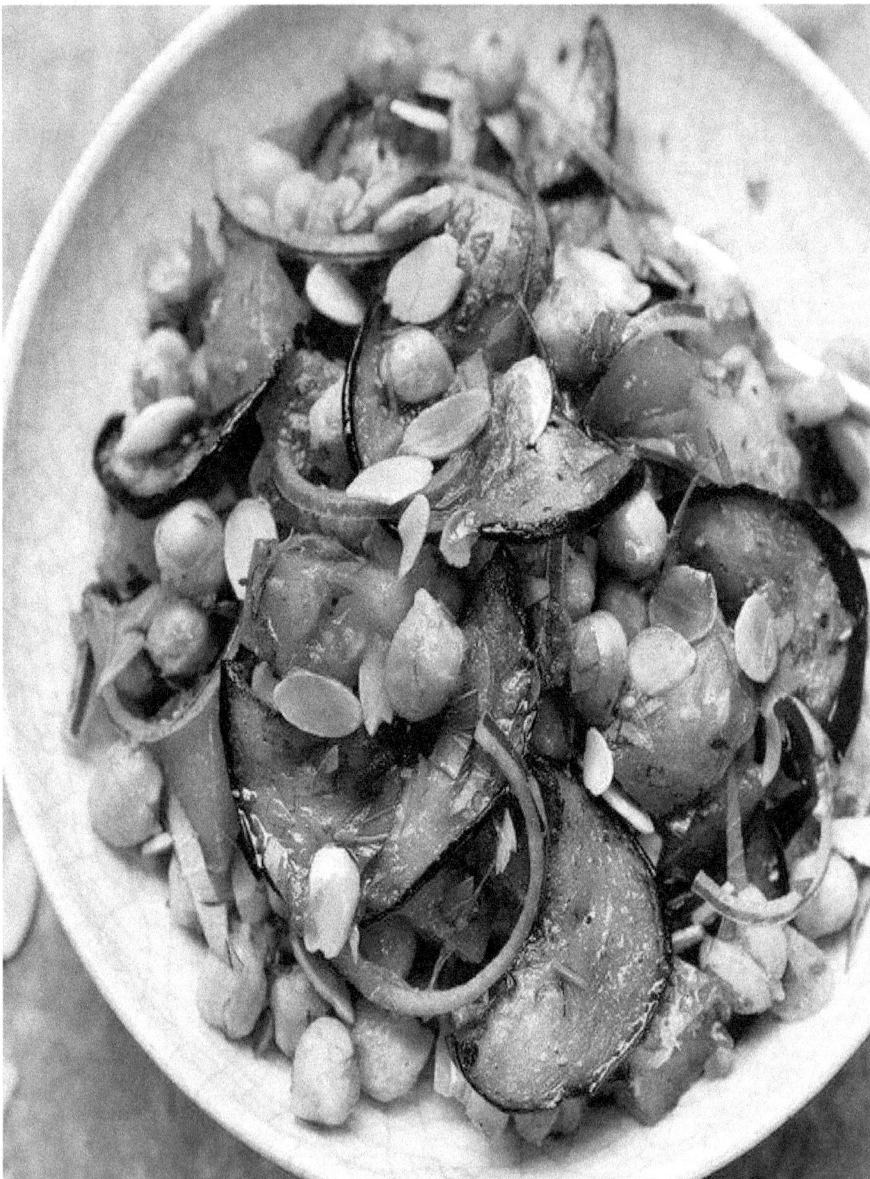

Prep time:

5 minutes | Cook time: 20 minutes | Serves 6

Ingredients

2 tablespoons freshly squeezed lemon juice

1 teaspoon ground cumin

¼ teaspoon sea salt

2 tablespoons olive oil, divided

1 (1-pound / 454-g) medium globe eggplant, stem removed, cut into flat cubes (about ½ inch thick)

2 tablespoons balsamic vinegar

1 (15-ounce / 425-g) can chickpeas, drained and rinsed

¼ cup chopped mint leaves

1 cup sliced sweet onion

1 garlic clove, finely minced

1 tablespoon sesame seeds, toasted

Direction

1. Preheat the oven to 550°F (288°C) or the highest level of your oven or broiler. Grease a baking sheet with 1 tablespoon of olive oil.
2. Combine the balsamic vinegar, lemon juice, cumin, salt, and 1 tablespoon of olive oil in a small bowl. Stir to mix well.
3. Arrange the eggplant cubes on the baking sheet, then brush with 2 tablespoons of the balsamic vinegar mixture on both sides.
4. Broil in the preheated oven for 8 minutes or until lightly browned. Flip the cubes halfway through the cooking time.
5. Meanwhile, combine the chickpeas, mint, onion, garlic, and sesame seeds in a large serving bowl. Drizzle with remaining balsamic vinegar mixture. Stir to mix well.
6. Remove the eggplant from the oven. Allow to cool for 5 minutes, then slice them into ½-inch strips on a clean work surface.
7. Add the eggplant strips in the serving bowl, then toss to combine well before serving.

Per Serving

Calories: 125 | fat: 2.9g | protein: 5.2g | carbs: 20.9g | fiber: 6.0g | sodium: 222mg

Italian Sautéd Cannellini Beans

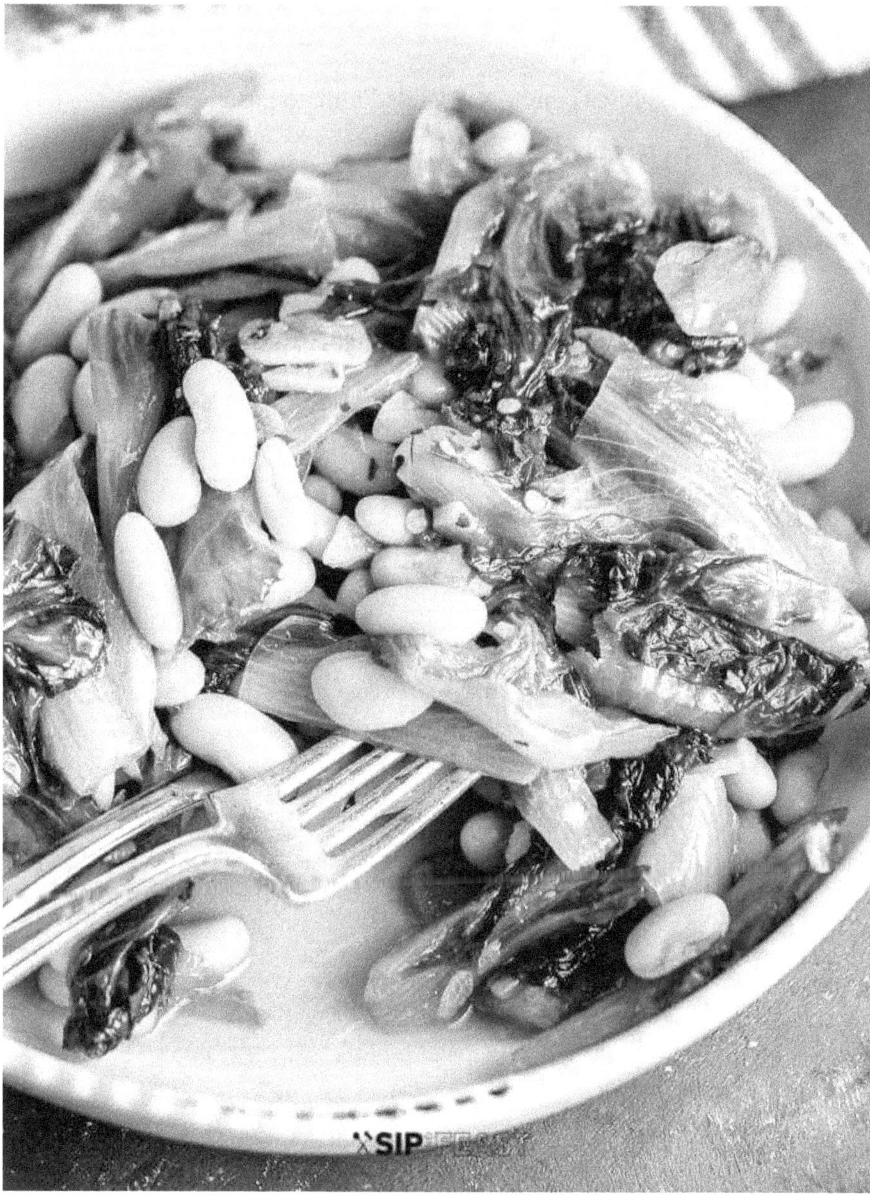

Prep time:

10 minutes | Cook time: 15 minutes | Serves 6

Ingredients

2 teaspoons extra-virgin olive oil

½ cup minced onion

¼ cup red wine vinegar

1 (12-ounce / 340-g) can no-salt-added tomato paste

2 tablespoons raw honey

½ cup water

¼ teaspoon ground cinnamon

Direction

1. 2 (15-ounce / 425-g) cans cannellini beans

1. Heat the olive oil in a saucepan over medium heat until shimmering.
2. Add the onion and sauté for 5 minutes or until translucent.
3. Pour in the red wine vinegar, tomato paste, honey, and water. Sprinkle with cinnamon. Stir to mix well.
4. Reduce the heat to low, then pour all the beans into the saucepan. Cook for 10 more minutes. Stir constantly.
5. Serve immediately.

Per Serving

Calories: 435 | fat: 2.1g | protein: 26.2g | carbs: 80.3g | fiber: 24.0g | sodium: 72mg

Lentil and Vegetable Curry Stew

Prep time:

20 minutes | Cook time: 4 hours 7 minutes | Serves 8

Ingredients

1 tablespoon coconut oil

1 yellow onion, diced

¼ cup yellow Thai curry paste

2 cups unsweetened coconut milk

2 cups dry red lentils, rinsed well and drained

3 cups bite-sized cauliflower florets

2 golden potatoes, cut into chunks

2 carrots, peeled and diced

8 cups low-sodium vegetable soup, divided

1 bunch kale, stems removed and roughly chopped

Sea salt, to taste

½ cup fresh cilantro, chopped

Pinch crushed red pepper flakes

Direction

1. Heat the coconut oil in a nonstick skillet over medium-high heat until melted.
2. Add the onion and sauté for 5 minutes or until translucent.
3. Pour in the curry paste and sauté for another 2 minutes, then fold in the coconut milk and stir to combine well. Bring to a simmer and turn off the heat.
4. Put the lentils, cauliflower, potatoes, and carrot in the slow cooker. Pour in 6 cups of vegetable soup and the curry mixture. Stir to combine well.
5. Cover and cook on high for 4 hours or until the lentils and vegetables are soft. Stir periodically.
6. During the last 30 minutes, fold the kale in the slow cooker and pour in the remaining vegetable soup. Sprinkle with salt.
7. Pour the stew in a large serving bowl and spread the cilantro and red pepper flakes on top before serving hot.

Per Serving

Calories: 530 | fat: 19.2g | protein: 20.3g | carbs: 75.2g | fiber: 15.5g | sodium: 562mg

Chickpea, Vegetable, and Fruit Stew

Prep time:

20 minutes | Cook time: 6 hours 4 minutes | Serves 6

Ingredients

1 large bell pepper, any color, chopped

6 ounces (170 g) green beans, trimmed and cut into bite-size pieces

3 cups canned chickpeas, rinsed and drained

1 (15-ounce / 425-g) can diced tomatoes, with the juice

1 large carrot, cut into ¼-inch rounds

2 large potatoes, peeled and cubed

1 large yellow onion, chopped

1 teaspoon grated fresh ginger

2 garlic cloves, minced

1¾ cups low-sodium vegetable soup

1 teaspoon ground cumin

1 tablespoon ground coriander

¼ teaspoon ground red pepper flakes

Sea salt and ground black pepper, to taste

8 ounces (227 g) fresh baby spinach

¼ cup diced dried figs

¼ cup diced dried apricots

1 cup plain Greek yogurt

Direction

1. Place the bell peppers, green beans, chicken peas, tomatoes and juice, carrot, potatoes, onion, ginger, and garlic in the slow cooker.
2. Pour in the vegetable soup and sprinkle with cumin, coriander, red pepper flakes, salt, and ground black pepper. Stir to mix well.
3. Put the slow cooker lid on and cook on high for 6 hours or until the vegetables are soft. Stir periodically.
4. Open the lid and fold in the spinach, figs, apricots, and yogurt. Stir to mix well.
5. Cook for 4 minutes or until the spinach is wilted. Pour them in a large serving bowl. Allow to cool for at least 20 minutes, then serve warm.

Per Serving

Calories: 611 | fat: 9.0g | protein: 30.7g | carbs: 107.4g | fiber: 20.8g | sodium: 344mg

Quinoa and Chickpea Vegetable Bowls

Prep time:

20 minutes | Cook time: 15 minutes | Serves 4

Ingredients

1 cup red dry quinoa, rinsed and drained

2 cups low-sodium vegetable soup

2 cups fresh spinach

2 cups finely shredded red cabbage

1 (15-ounce / 425-g) can chickpeas, drained and rinsed

1 ripe avocado, thinly sliced

1 cup shredded carrots

1 red bell pepper, thinly sliced

4 tablespoons Mango Sauce

½ cup fresh cilantro, chopped

Mango Sauce:

1 mango, diced

¼ cup fresh lime juice

½ teaspoon ground turmeric

1 teaspoon finely minced fresh ginger

¼ teaspoon sea salt

Pinch of ground red pepper

1 teaspoon pure maple syrup

2 tablespoons extra-virgin olive oil

Direction

1. Pour the quinoa and vegetable soup in a saucepan. Bring to a boil. Reduce the heat to low. Cover and cook for 15 minutes or until tender. Fluffy with a fork.
2. Meanwhile, combine the **Ingredients** for the mango sauce in a food processor. Pulse until smooth.
3. Divide the quinoa, spinach, and cabbage into 4 serving bowls, then top with chickpeas, avocado, carrots, and bell pepper. Dress them with the mango sauce and spread with cilantro. Serve immediately.

Per Serving

Calories: 366 | fat: 11.1g | protein: 15.5g | carbs: 55.6g | fiber: 17.7g | sodium: 746mg

Ritzy Veggie Chili

Prep time:

15 minutes | Cook time: 5 hours | Serves 4

Ingredients

1 (28-ounce / 794-g) can chopped tomatoes, with the juice

1 (15-ounce / 425-g) can black beans, drained and rinsed

1 (15-ounce / 425-g) can redly beans, drained and rinsed

1 medium green bell pepper, chopped

1 yellow onion, chopped

1 tablespoon onion powder

1 teaspoon paprika

1 teaspoon cayenne pepper

1 teaspoon garlic powder

½ teaspoon sea salt

½ teaspoon ground black pepper

1 tablespoon olive oil

1 large hass avocado, pitted, peeled, and chopped, for garnish

Direction

1. Combine all the **Ingredients,** except for the avocado, in the slow cooker. Stir to mix well.
2. Put the slow cooker lid on and cook on high for 5 hours or until the vegetables are tender and the mixture has a thick consistency.
3. Pour the chili in a large serving bowl. Allow to cool for 30 minutes, then spread with chopped avocado and serve.

Per Serving

Calories: 633 | fat: 16.3g | protein: 31.7g | carbs: 97.0g | fiber: 28.9g | sodium: 792mg

Spicy Italian Bean Balls with Marinara

Prep time:

20 minutes | Cook time: 30 minutes | Serves 2 to 4

Ingredients

Bean Balls:

1 tablespoon extra-virgin olive oil

½ yellow onion, minced

1 teaspoon fennel seeds

2 teaspoons dried oregano

½ teaspoon crushed red pepper flakes

1 teaspoon garlic powder

1 (15-ounce / 425-g) can white beans (cannellini or navy), drained and rinsed

½ cup whole-grain bread crumbs

Sea salt and ground black pepper, to taste

Marinara:

1 tablespoon extra-virgin olive oil

3 garlic cloves, minced

Handful basil leaves

1 (28-ounce / 794-g) can chopped tomatoes with juice reserved

Sea salt, to taste

Direction

Make the Bean Balls

1. Preheat the oven to 350°F (180°C). Line a baking sheet with parchment paper.
2. Heat the olive oil in a nonstick skillet over medium heat until shimmering.
3. Add the onion and sauté for 5 minutes or until translucent.
4. Sprinkle with fennel seeds, oregano, red pepper flakes, and garlic powder, then cook for 1 minute or until aromatic.
5. Pour the sautéed mixture in a food processor and add the beans and bread crumbs. Sprinkle with salt and ground black pepper, then pulse to combine well and the mixture holds together.
6. Shape the mixture into balls with a 2-ounce (57-g) cookie scoop, then arrange the balls on the baking sheet.
7. Bake in the preheated oven for 30 minutes or until lightly browned. Flip the balls halfway through the cooking time.

Make the Marinara

8. While baking the bean balls, heat the olive oil in a saucepan over medium-high heat until shimmering.
9. Add the garlic and basil and sauté for 2 minutes or until fragrant.
10. Fold in the tomatoes and juice. Bring to a boil. Reduce the heat to low. Put the lid on and simmer for 15 minutes. Sprinkle with salt.
11. Transfer the bean balls on a large plate and baste with marinara before serving.

Per Serving

Calories: 351 | fat: 16.4g | protein: 11.5g | carbs: 42.9g | fiber: 10.3g | sodium: 377mg

Wild Rice, Celery, and Cauliflower Pilaf

Prep time:

10 minutes | Cook time: 45 minutes | Serves 4

Ingredients

1 tablespoon olive oil, plus more for greasing the baking dish

1 cup wild rice

2 cups low-sodium chicken broth

1 sweet onion, chopped

2 stalks celery, chopped

1 teaspoon minced garlic

2 carrots, peeled, halved lengthwise, and sliced

½ cauliflower head, cut into small florets

1 teaspoon chopped fresh thyme

Sea salt, to taste

Direction

1. Preheat the oven to 350°F (180°C). Line a baking sheet with parchment paper and grease with olive oil.
2. Put the wild rice in a saucepan, then pour in the chicken broth. Bring to a boil. Reduce the heat to low and simmer for 30 minutes or until the rice is plump.
3. Meanwhile, heat the remaining olive oil in an oven-proof skillet over medium-high heat until shimmering.
4. Add the onion, celery, and garlic to the skillet and sauté for 3 minutes or until the onion is translucent.
5. Add the carrots and cauliflower to the skillet and sauté for 5 minutes. Turn off the heat and set aside.
6. Pour the cooked rice in the skillet with the vegetables. Sprinkle with thyme and salt.
7. Set the skillet in the preheated oven and bake for 15 minutes or until the vegetables are soft.
8. Serve immediately.

Per Serving

Calories: 214 | fat: 3.9g | protein: 7.2g | carbs: 37.9g | fiber: 5.0g | sodium: 122mg

Walnut and Ricotta Spaghetti

Prep time:

15 minutes | Cook time: 10 minutes | Serves 6

Ingredients

1 pound (454 g) cooked whole-wheat spaghetti

2 tablespoons extra-virgin olive oil

4 cloves garlic, minced

¾ cup walnuts, toasted and finely chopped

2 tablespoons ricotta cheese

¼ cup flat-leaf parsley, chopped

½ cup grated Parmesan cheese

Sea salt and freshly ground pepper, to taste

Direction

1. Reserve a cup of spaghetti water while cooking the spaghetti.
2. Heat the olive oil in a nonstick skillet over medium-low heat or until shimmering.
3. Add the garlic and sauté for a minute or until fragrant.
4. Pour the spaghetti water into the skillet and cook for 8 more minutes.
5. Turn off the heat and mix in the walnuts and ricotta cheese.
6. Put the cooked spaghetti on a large serving plate, then pour the walnut sauce over. Spread with parsley and Parmesan, then sprinkle with salt and ground pepper. Toss to serve.

Per Serving

Calories: 264 | fat: 16.8g | protein: 8.6g | carbs: 22.8g | fiber: 4.0g | sodium: 336mg

Butternut Squash, Spinach, and Cheeses Lasagna

Prep time:

30 minutes | Cook time: 3 hours 45 minutes | Serves 4 to 6

Ingredients

2 tablespoons extra-virgin olive oil, divided

1 butternut squash, halved lengthwise and deseeded

½ teaspoon sage

½ teaspoon sea salt

¼ teaspoon ground black pepper

¼ cup grated Parmesan cheese

2 cups ricotta cheese

½ cup unsweetened almond milk

5 layers whole-wheat lasagna noodles (about 12 ounces / 340 g in total)

4 ounces (113 g) fresh spinach leaves, divided

½ cup shredded part skim Mozzarella, for garnish

Direction

1. Preheat the oven to 400°F (205°C). Line a baking sheet with parchment paper.
2. Brush 1 tablespoon of olive oil on the cut side of the butternut squash, then place the squash on the baking sheet.
3. Bake in the preheated oven for 45 minutes or until the squash is tender.
4. Allow to cool until you can handle it, then scoop the flesh out and put the flesh in a food processor to purée.
5. Combine the puréed butternut squash flesh with sage, salt, and ground black pepper in a large bowl. Stir to mix well.
6. Combine the cheeses and milk in a separate bowl, then sprinkle with salt and pepper, to taste.
7. Grease the slow cooker with 1 tablespoon of olive oil, then add a layer of lasagna noodles to coat the bottom of the slow cooker.
8. Spread half of the squash mixture on top of the noodles, then top the squash mixture with another layer of lasagna noodles.
9. Spread half of the spinach over the noodles, then top the spinach with half of cheese mixture. Repeat with remaining 3 layers of lasagna noodles, squash mixture, spinach, and cheese mixture.
10. Top the cheese mixture with Mozzarella, then put the lid on and cook on low for 3 hours or until the lasagna noodles are al dente.
11. Serve immediately.

Per Serving

Calories: 657 | fat: 37.1g | protein: 30.9g | carbs: 57.2g | fiber: 8.3g | sodium: 918mg

Minestrone Chickpeas and Macaroni Casserole

Prep time:

20 minutes | Cook time: 7 hours 20 minutes | Serves 5

Ingredients

1 (15-ounce / 425-g) can chickpeas, drained and rinsed

1 (28-ounce / 794-g) can diced tomatoes, with the juice

1 (6-ounce / 170-g) can no-salt-added tomato paste

3 medium carrots, sliced

3 cloves garlic, minced

1 medium yellow onion, chopped

1 cup low-sodium vegetable soup

½ teaspoon dried rosemary

1 teaspoon dried oregano

2 teaspoons maple syrup

½ teaspoon sea salt

¼ teaspoon ground black pepper

½ pound (227-g) fresh green beans, trimmed and cut into bite-size pieces

1 cup macaroni pasta

2 ounces (57 g) Parmesan cheese, grated

Direction

1. Except for the green beans, pasta, and Parmesan cheese, combine all the **Ingredients** in the slow cooker and stir to mix well.
2. Put the slow cooker lid on and cook on low for 7 hours.
3. Fold in the pasta and green beans. Put the lid on and cook on high for 20 minutes or until the vegetable are soft and the pasta is al dente.
4. Pour them in a large serving bowl and spread with Parmesan cheese before serving.

Per Serving

Calories: 349 | fat: 6.7g | protein: 16.5g | carbs: 59.9g | fiber: 12.9g | sodium: 937mg

Garlic and Parsley Chickpeas

Prep time:

10 minutes | Cook time: 18 to 20 minutes | Serves 4 to 6

Ingredients

¼ cup extra-virgin olive oil, divided

4 garlic cloves, sliced thinly

⅛ teaspoon red pepper flakes

1 onion, chopped finely

¼ teaspoon salt, plus more to taste

Black pepper, to taste

2 (15-ounce / 425-g) cans chickpeas, rinsed

1 cup vegetable broth

2 tablespoons minced fresh parsley

2 teaspoons lemon juice

Direction

1. Add 3 tablespoons of the olive oil, garlic, and pepper flakes to a skillet over medium heat. Cook for about 3 minutes, stirring constantly, or until the garlic turns golden but not brown.
2. Stir in the onion and ¼ teaspoon salt and cook for 5 to 7 minutes, or until softened and lightly browned.
3. Add the chickpeas and broth to the skillet and bring to a simmer. Reduce the heat to medium-low, cover, and cook for about 7 minutes, or until the chickpeas are cooked through and flavors meld.
4. Uncover, increase the heat to high and continue to cook for about 3 minutes more, or until nearly all liquid has evaporated.
5. Turn off the heat, stir in the parsley and lemon juice. Season to taste with salt and pepper and drizzle with remaining 1 tablespoon of the olive oil.
6. Serve warm.

Per Serving

Calories: 220 | fat: 11.4g | protein: 6.5g | carbs: 24.6g | fiber: 6.0g | sodium: 467mg

Black-Eyed Peas Salad with Walnuts

Prep time:

10 minutes | Cook time: 0 minutes | Serves 4 to 6

Ingredients

3 tablespoons extra-virgin olive oil

3 tablespoons dukkah, divided

2 tablespoons lemon juice

2 tablespoons pomegranate molasses

¼ teaspoon salt, or more to taste

⅛ teaspoon pepper, or more to taste

2 (15-ounce / 425-g) cans black-eyed peas, rinsed

½ cup pomegranate seeds

½ cup minced fresh parsley

½ cup walnuts, toasted and chopped

4 scallions, sliced thinly

Direction

1. In a large bowl, whisk together the olive oil, 2 tablespoons of the dukkah, lemon juice, pomegranate molasses, salt and pepper.
2. Stir in the remaining **Ingredients**. Season with salt and pepper.
3. Sprinkle with the remaining 1 tablespoon of the dukkah before serving.

Per Serving

Calories: 155 | fat: 11.5g | protein: 2.0g | carbs: 12.5g | fiber: 2.1g | sodium: 105mg

Mashed Beans with Cumin

Prep time:

10 minutes | Cook time: 10 to 12 minutes | Serves 4 to 6

Ingredients

1 tablespoon extra-virgin olive oil, plus extra for serving

4 garlic cloves, minced

1 teaspoon ground cumin

2 (15-ounce / 425-g) cans fava beans

3 tablespoons tahini

2 tablespoons lemon juice, plus lemon wedges for serving

Salt and pepper, to taste

1 tomato, cored and cut into ½-inch pieces

1 small onion, chopped finely

2 hard-cooked large eggs, chopped

2 tablespoons minced fresh parsley

Direction

1. Add the olive oil, garlic and cumin to a medium saucepan over medium heat. Cook for about 2 minutes, or until fragrant.
2. Stir in the beans with their liquid and tahini. Bring to a simmer and cook for 8 to 10 minutes, or until the liquid thickens slightly.
3. Turn off the heat, mash the beans to a coarse consistency with a potato masher. Stir in the lemon juice and 1 teaspoon pepper. Season with salt and pepper.
4. Transfer the mashed beans to a serving dish. Top with the tomato, onion, eggs and parsley. Drizzle with the extra olive oil.
5. Serve with the lemon wedges.

Per Serving

Calories: 125 | fat: 8.6g | protein: 4.9g | carbs: 9.1g | fiber: 2.9g | sodium: 131mg

Turkish Canned Pinto Bean Salad

Prep time:

10 minutes | Cook time: 3 minutes | Serves 4 to 6

Ingredients

¼ cup extra-virgin olive oil, divided

3 garlic cloves, lightly crushed and peeled

2 (15-ounce / 425-g) cans pinto beans, rinsed 2 cups plus

1 tablespoon water

Salt and pepper, to taste

¼ cup tahini

3 tablespoons lemon juice

1 tablespoon ground dried Aleppo pepper, plus extra for serving

8 ounces (227 g) cherry tomatoes, halved

¼ red onion, sliced thinly

½ cup fresh parsley leaves

2 hard-cooked large eggs, quartered

1 tablespoon toasted sesame seeds

Direction

1. Add 1 tablespoon of the olive oil and garlic to a medium saucepan over medium heat. Cook for about 3 minutes, stirring constantly, or until the garlic turns golden but not brown.
2. Add the beans, 2 cups of the water and 1 teaspoon salt and bring to a simmer. Remove from the heat, cover and let sit for 20 minutes. Drain the beans and discard the garlic.
3. In a large bowl, whisk together the remaining 3 tablespoons of the oil, tahini, lemon juice, Aleppo, the remaining 1 tablespoon of the water and ¼ teaspoon salt. Stir in the beans, tomatoes, onion and parsley. Season with salt and pepper to taste.
4. Transfer to a serving platter and top with the eggs. Sprinkle with the sesame seeds and extra Aleppo before serving.

Per Serving

Calories: 402 | fat: 18.9g | protein: 16.2g | carbs: 44.4g | fiber: 11.2g | sodium: 456mg

Fava and Garbanzo Bean Ful

Prep time:

10 minutes | Cook time: 10 minutes | Serves 6

Ingredients

1 (15-ounce / 425-g) can fava beans, rinsed and drained

1 (1-pound / 454-g) can garbanzo beans, rinsed and drained

3 cups water

½ cup lemon juice

3 cloves garlic, peeled and minced

1 teaspoon salt

3 tablespoons extra-virgin olive oil

Direction

1. In a pot over medium heat, cook the beans and water for 10 minutes.
2. Drain the beans and transfer to a bowl. Reserve 1 cup of the liquid from the cooked beans.
3. Add the reserved liquid, lemon juice, minced garlic and salt to the bowl with the beans. Mix to combine well. Using a potato masher, mash up about half the beans in the bowl.
4. Give the mixture one more stir to make sure the beans are evenly mixed.
5. Drizzle with the olive oil and serve.

Per Serving

Calories: 199 | fat: 9.0g | protein: 10.0g | carbs: 25.0g | fiber: 9.0g | sodium: 395mg

Triple-Green Pasta with Cheese

Prep time:

5 minutes | Cook time: 14 to 16 minutes | Serves 4

Ingredients

8 ounces (227 g) uncooked penne

1 tablespoon extra-virgin olive oil

2 garlic cloves, minced

¼ teaspoon crushed red pepper

2 cups chopped fresh flat-leaf parsley, including stems

5 cups loosely packed baby spinach

¼ teaspoon ground nutmeg

¼ teaspoon kosher salt

¼ teaspoon freshly ground black pepper

⅓ cup Castelvetrano olives, pitted and sliced

⅓ cup grated Parmesan cheese

Direction

1. In a large stockpot of salted water, cook the pasta for about 8 to 10 minutes. Drain the pasta and reserve ¼ cup of the cooking liquid.
2. Meanwhile, heat the olive oil in a large skillet over medium heat. Add the garlic and red pepper and cook for 30 seconds, stirring constantly.
3. Add the parsley and cook for 1 minute, stirring constantly. Add the spinach, nutmeg, salt, and pepper, and cook for 3 minutes, stirring occasionally, or until the spinach is wilted.
4. Add the cooked pasta and the reserved ¼ cup cooking liquid to the skillet. Stir in the olives and cook for about 2 minutes, or until most of the pasta water has been absorbed.
5. Remove from the heat and stir in the cheese before serving.

Per Serving

Calories: 262 | fat: 4.0g | protein: 15.0g | carbs: 51.0g | fiber: 13.0g | sodium: 1180mg

Caprese Pasta with Roasted Asparagus

Prep time:

5 minutes | Cook time: 25 minutes | Serves 6

Ingredients

8 ounces (227 g) uncooked small pasta, like orecchiette (little ears) or farfalle (bow ties)

1½ pounds (680 g) fresh asparagus, ends trimmed and stalks chopped into 1-inch pieces

1½ cups grape tomatoes, halved

2 tablespoons extra-virgin olive oil

¼ teaspoon kosher salt

¼ teaspoon freshly ground black pepper

2 cups fresh Mozzarella, drained and cut into bite-size pieces (about 8 ounces / 227 g)

⅓ cup torn fresh basil leaves

2 tablespoons balsamic vinegar

Direction

1. Preheat the oven to 400ºF (205ºC).
2. In a large stockpot of salted water, cook the pasta for about 8 to 10 minutes. Drain and reserve about ¼ cup of the cooking liquid.
3. Meanwhile, in a large bowl, toss together the asparagus, tomatoes, oil, salt and pepper. Spread the mixture onto a large, rimmed baking sheet and bake in the oven for 15 minutes, stirring twice during cooking.
4. Remove the vegetables from the oven and add the cooked pasta to the baking sheet. Mix with a few tablespoons of cooking liquid to help the sauce become smoother and the saucy vegetables stick to the pasta.
5. Gently mix in the Mozzarella and basil. Drizzle with the balsamic vinegar. Serve from the baking sheet or pour the pasta into a large bowl.

Per Serving

Calories: 147 | fat: 3.0g | protein: 16.0g | carbs: 17.0g | fiber: 5.0g | sodium: 420mg

Alphabetical Index

CPSIA information can be obtained
at www.ICGtesting.com
Printed in the USA
BVHW080224190521
607644BV00013B/1369

9 781802 837704